Maite Concepción Hernández
Silvia Beatriz Garay Cruz
Omelio Cepero Rodríguez

Homeopathy in stomatology

Maite Concepción Hernández
Silvia Beatriz Garay Cruz
Omelio Cepero Rodríguez

Homeopathy in stomatology

Homeopathic drugs in stomatology, treatment of stomatologic diseases and affections

ScienciaScripts

Imprint

Any brand names and product names mentioned in this book are subject to trademark, brand or patent protection and are trademarks or registered trademarks of their respective holders. The use of brand names, product names, common names, trade names, product descriptions etc. even without a particular marking in this work is in no way to be construed to mean that such names may be regarded as unrestricted in respect of trademark and brand protection legislation and could thus be used by anyone.

Cover image: www.ingimage.com

This book is a translation from the original published under ISBN 978-620-3-03151-5.

Publisher:
Sciencia Scripts
is a trademark of
Dodo Books Indian Ocean Ltd. and OmniScriptum S.R.L publishing group

120 High Road, East Finchley, London, N2 9ED, United Kingdom
Str. Armeneasca 28/1, office 1, Chisinau MD-2012, Republic of Moldova, Europe
Managing Directors: Ieva Konstantinova, Victoria Ursu
info@omniscriptum.com

Printed at: see last page
ISBN: 978-620-3-40359-6

Summary

Homeopathy is a therapeutic system that uses natural medicines whose objective is to cure according to the laws of healing. It was created by Hahneman more than 200 years ago and is based on the principle of similarity, an ancient principle proposed by Hippocrates and put into practice by Hahneman, which recognizes the body's ability to heal itself and states that the disease can be cured by substances capable of causing a condition or symptom similar to that of the disease to be treated. The therapy based on these principles is fundamentally characterized by being non-invasive, low cost, uses non-toxic remedies, can be used in acute and chronic disorders, and is essentially holistic, since it considers the patient in his emotional, mental and physical level, aiming to restore the lost balance. Homeopathic remedies are obtained from plants, minerals and animals. These medicines can be administered in drops, globules and tablets. They can be applied on the tongue, sublingually, on the lips, by inhalation or taken in solutions. In stomatology, this science offers us multiple advantages and benefits with minimal side effects: cost savings and the opening of a new line of research and treatment.

Keywords: Homeopathy; Stomatology; Stomatologic diseases.
Homeopathic Pharmacology.

Table of Contents

Introduction

The use of alternative medicine such as homeopathy, traditional Chinese medicine, although it has existed for a long time and was for many years the first therapeutic choice for people's ailments, was relegated by doctors and patients in favor of modern medicine, as the success and renown achieved by the latter grew.

These successes achieved by modern medicine derived from the possibility of making increasingly specific diagnoses of strange and complicated pathologies; of providing specific treatment for pathologies such as infections, cancer, inflammatory diseases; and in terms of public health, from the reduction of indicators such as prevalence, incidence, mortality and lethality rates, etc., and allowed this modern conception of medicine to be adopted by the health systems of industrialized countries and by dragging developing countries along with it, and to become the hegemonic medical model.

These complications, together with an integrative vision of the human being and the desire to return to nature as the source of health, have allowed people to look again to alternative medicines as their first therapeutic option.

In the specific case of homeopathy, it has been successfully used since the 18th century in the management of acute and chronic pathologies, considering in this management the physical and mental symptoms of the disease as a whole and therefore looking at the patient as a whole.

It is precisely this integrative management of the symptoms and the patient that allows us to assume that the use of homeopathy is adequate for the management of a pathology as widespread in humanity and with as many risk factors as hypertension.

Homeopathy is a way of healing, since it is not the homeopathic medicine that cures, but the patient who heals himself, under the stimulus of the remedy, which sets in motion the individual's own healing mechanisms, conditioned only by the vitality of the patient, that is, the homeopathic medicine works as an organic stimulator, which does not act in isolated organs, nor has the same manifestation or response in all individuals (Silva, 1994). It takes the sick individual and treats his disturbances in the physical, emotional and mental planes at the same time. It manages to restore the lost balance of the sick individual at the three levels, through the stimulation and reinforcement of its defense mechanism (autoimmune system, reticuloendothelial system, hormonal system, sympathetic-parasympathetic system and the psychological mechanism that responds to stress) (Vithoukas, 1989).

In 1798, Hahnemann stated: *"If the Law of Medicine is recognized and proclaimed as real, true and natural, it must find its application of homeopathy in animals"*, by applying this therapy to his own horse (Sanchez, 1994).

Homeopathy is not an alternative or complementary medicine, since it is a medical system that has been studied, researched and applied for more than 200 years, and has its own doctrine that has been widely proven. It is considered official medicine in England, France, Spain, Cuba and many countries around the world, which even have exclusively homeopathic hospitals (Cass and Chein, 1999).

This medical system, created by Hahnemann, is based on the Law of Similarity, which states that to cure a sick individual, a substance should be used that in a healthy individual has been able to produce a similar symptomatic picture to the one to be treated (Brand, 1994; Guajardo, 1994 and Ancarola, 1996).

It is a medical discipline which has its primary emphasis on therapy, being a low-cost system employing exclusively non-toxic drugs. It can be used to treat both acute and chronic cases, but its magnificent contribution lies in its successful treatment of chronic diseases, which have become difficult to manage by orthodox methods (Hunter, 1996 and Robinson, 1996). There is an important fundamental difference between homeopathy and other therapeutics, and that is that it treats patients and not diseases, hence the decisive importance of individualization (Muratas, 1990 and Edwards, 1995).

The objective of this work is to show the possible homeopathic medicines to be used in the treatment of different stomatological emergencies, taking into account the way each patient suffers from these conditions.

Homeopathy. Concept, history and distribution

The word homeopathy comes from the Greek: Homois, similar; and Pathos, suffering. The system created by Hahnemann caught the attention of a Londoner, Dr. Frederick Hervey Foster Quin, who became a convinced homeopath and was the first president of the British Homeopathic Society from 1844 until his death in 1878. Correspondents from Canada noted that the average age at which homeopathic physicians die is twenty years older than that of their allopathic colleagues.

Human and animal diseases were treated without rational and logical principles, but according to various esoteric, hypothetical, curative paradigms in which the palliative rule was: contraria, contrariis, curentur. The truth is actually diametrically opposite: to cure medium, fast and permanently in every disorder, select the medicine which produces a similar clinical picture: simila, similibus, curentur. This is the main foundation of Flomeopathy (known as the Law of Cure).

Homeopathic therapies are not at odds with other medical specialties and obviously surgical, orthopedic, psychiatric and intensive care activities are essential for the solution of certain conditions in patients.

Homeopathy is a way of healing, since it is not the homeopathic medicine that cures, but the patient, under the stimulus of the remedy (stimulates the bioenergetic capacity), which sets in motion the healing mechanisms of the individual, conditioned only by the vitality of the patient, that is, the homeopathic medicine works as an organic stimulator, which does not act in isolated organs, nor has the same manifestation or response in all individuals.

This medicine is based on a set of basic laws or principles such as: The Law of Similars. Law of Proofs. Law of the Simple Remedy. Law of the Minimum Dose and the Theory of the dynamization of the medicine (potency). Law of the Direction of the Cure and the Law of the Doctrine of the Miasms.

The law of similars

This law forms the key to homeopathic practice. The bases that allowed Hahnemann to formulate this law were the following:

That any symptom complex or syndrome is not the disease as such, but the defense action mechanism mobilized by the body in contact with an influence is what causes the disease, being this a specific stress such as a bacterium or a virus, or a non-specific stress such as climate changes, environmental pollution, emotional or mental disturbances, among others.

The symptoms do not constitute the disease, but the reactions of the organism under stress are the means by which the organism attempts against its lost physiological balance (homeostasis).

An organized system in equilibrium responds to any particular disturbance force at the optimum time.

To help the organism restore its order, the physician should assist and reinforce these reactions rather than suppress them. The correct homeopathic remedy is chosen by assuming that the patient is extremely receptive to that particular remedy and only that specific remedy, which is capable of producing his symptomatology. "Simila Similibus Curentur" can be explained as the same substance capable of producing the specific symptoms in a healthy individual, can cure a patient of a disease by producing identical or similar symptoms.

Suppression of symptoms (known as contrapathy or antipathy) is one of the major dangers of allopathic medicine. The contraria (contraris) paradigm is used in Oriental medicine to oppose the symptoms of disease.

The Law of Evidence

Hahnemann experimented on groups of healthy human volunteers, including himself, by orally taking medicinal plants, minerals and animal substances. He found that when active medicinal materials are ingested by humans in sufficient quantity, they produce a pattern of symptoms, which more often than not, initiate a natural disease, either acute or chronic.

The Law of the Single Remedy
The one who wishes to perform an ultimate cure on the patient must prescribe one and only one specific remedy that has produced in his tests, the closest similarity to the symptom complex present in a patient. Any other remedy will have no real curative effect.

The single remedy has the advantage that when a remedy is administered one can evaluate its action. However, if some are administered, one cannot evaluate or know which one cured, or in what proportion.

This is known as individualization. However, there are many remedies that have a broad spectrum of action, these are employed when the disease exhibits diverse and sometimes vague symptomatology. Other groups of patients show common characteristics. Remedies known as constitutional are used in these cases.

The Law of Minimum Dose (homeopathic dose)

When homeopathy found the relevant individual remedy, the specific allergen to which an allergic person was sensitive was discovered. It is understood by this that in homeopathy the homeopath has to prescribe a very small dose, in order not to cause an enormous aggravation of the patient's symptomatology.

This law is compatible with the Arnolt-Schultz Law, which states that small doses stimulate, medium doses paralyze and large doses kill. According to this law, the action of small and very large doses of the same substance of living matter is opposite. Under this law comes the whole question of potency. After the initial microdoses have acted on the patient, it will bring a healing response through a cascading sequence of internal events, such as the reinforcement of defense mechanisms, re-establishing the vital balance with the organism. In this way, the remedy acts as a catalytic agent and usually does not need to be repeated frequently. In addition, the pharmaceutical cost of homeopathic treatment is lower.

The initial aggravation of the patient's symptoms is followed by a total improvement which, together with the observation of the Law of Cure, is a confirmation that an ultimate repair of health has taken place and not a suppression.

Law of the Direction of the Cure.
The reestablishment of internal order and the consequent return to health of the sick individual was observed to follow a predictable pattern. In the progressive march of symptoms as the cure occurs, it is noted that the main symptomatology moves from the most vital to the less vital functional centers within the organism. In other words, from the vital organs to the skin and from the mental to the emotional and finally to the physical. In the healing process, the rapid reappearance of old symptoms is also noted as a residue of the previous suppressed disease, making its way to the periphery to be eliminated by the homeopathically reinforced defense. By giving the actual medicine simillium, the symptoms are cured according to Hering's four laws. As in all holistic therapies and natural healing systems, the process involves an initial aggravation of the symptom as a defense mechanism. In a successful homeopathic treatment the initial elimination phase with the average presentation of symptoms is quickly followed by an improvement of all symptoms and return to normal health. The cure is considered complete when there is a total reestablishment of normal vital functions, expressed as optimal function of the mental, emotional and physical spheres of life.

The Doctrine of the Miasmas.

This was Hahnemann's hypothesis to explain many disorders, which seemed to be based on hereditary-familial treatises. Hahnemann classified them as Psora, Psychosis and Syphilis. This demonstrates his ingenuity in discussing genetics and transmissible disorders at a time before Mendel, when little was understood on this subject, which produced the admission that each disease was unique and individual, but can occur in common. The basic fundamentals of homeopathy include:

The dynamic and immaterial conception of illness and healing.

The profound knowledge of the capacity of a dynamized substance to modify the equilibrium of the state of health of a healthy man, as a prerequisite for its subsequent application as a medicine for the cure of an individual case of disease.

The application of the natural law of analogy in the art of healing: Simila Similibus Curanthum (like cures like).

The only remedy to administer each time is the one of maximum analogy and doing it in a simple way, that is, without mixing or combining it.

The subtle dose of a well-dynamized homeopathic remedy.

As far as the diagnosis of the affected area is concerned, there is an important difference between homeopathy and other therapies, and that is that it treats patients and not diseases, hence the decisive importance of individualization.

Homeopathy: Suggestion or faith?

It has been suggested time and again that homeopathy is a kind of faith healing, but this is a very superficial judgment, since it also has a favorable impact on children and, in fact, often achieves more spectacular results with very young children, since their symptoms are not clouded by the use of a series of drugs, as is the case with the chronically ill.

Some of the results achieved with the animals are truly astonishing, and it cannot be said that the animals are suggestible or place great faith in those who prescribe the medicines. Some years ago on a chinchilla farm an epidemic of gastroenteritis broke out and two veterinarians came to the conclusion that all the animals had to be exterminated. A homeopath was called in and sent a packet of low potency Arsenicum album to be mixed in the chinchillas' drinking water, as the animals were continually thirsty. Those most affected died, but three quarters of the valuable chinchillas were saved.

The Scottish Express of December 17, 1967 told of the serious epidemic of foot and mouth disease that was ravaging the Chresire and Shropshire regions and how one hundred farmers were persuaded to administer borax to their cows as a preventative measure, as a result of which numerous head of cattle were saved. These are just two incidents in a lifetime of homeopathic practice, demonstrating that homeopathy is more than just healing by faith or suggestion.

Homeopathy: scientific discipline or fiction?

This therapy demonstrates its scientific character by meeting the parameters of repeatability, verification, experimentation, abstraction and generalization. At the international level, the following are cited

countries such as England, where a certification in homeopathy for primary health care was held for the first time in 1994 at the University of Glasgow. In Scotland, general practitioners have undergone training in homeopathy. In France, family physicians have incorporated homeopathy into their daily practice. Courses at different scientific levels on the use of this type of therapy have been given. A constant concern is to set aside metaphysical concepts and to take this therapy along the path of investigative methodology.

Homeopathy and allopathic medicine: the same or different?

There are four of Hahnemann's ideas that must be analyzed in order to understand the difference between Homeopathic and Allopathic Medicine.

The first idea, or mental image, of Hahnemann consists in thinking of the patient as an individual, as a trilogy formed by the body, the mind and the spirit; as well as that any treatment should be directed to help these three facets of the personality, each one of them with its own reactions and peculiarities.

His second idea consists in considering disease as a malaise or disharmony, which indicates a state of disorder in the person and not a label with which to define the various symptoms, signs and clinical findings.

His third idea is to consider drugs or medicines as means to restore harmony and not as lethal weapons to destroy bacilli and streptococci, which nature surely created for a better purpose than to be destroyed by human intelligence.

Finally, his fourth mental image consists of realizing that the body can maintain its own defenses against lethal weapons disguised as strong medication and that the patient's life force can, many times, oppose infections with its own mechanisms, such as fever which, if left alone, will be able to burn up any infection that presents itself.

Homeopathy seems to be most useful in treating chronic diseases and patients who do not respond to allopathic treatment. Remarkable recoveries have been reported in the treatment of chronic kidney disease, digestive abnormalities and old lameness. It is practiced all over the world, from Great Britain to Nepal. Its methods have often clashed with those of modern medicine because of diametrically opposed treatment philosophies.

What for allopathy is the cause of the disease, for homeopathy is a causative factor, another manifestation of the disease in a specific form and location. Homeopathic thinking is labyrinthine, it does not have the logic of the line, it is a path with obstacles as unpredictable as life is, perception makes us go slowly locating the right path, with great patience, until we find the right way out. In this model of thought everything can be joined to everything. For the principle of similarity what is above is comparable to what is below, what is below is comparable to what is above.

The advantages of Homeopathy over conventional medicine are:

Individualization of treatment in view of symptoms.

Absence of drug toxicity, avoiding the accumulation of toxic residues in slaughter animals and their production.

Application of this therapeutic in the new trends of animal production aimed at obtaining ecological productions.

Absence of side effects.

Ease of administration.

It helps to improve knowledge about people and our animals, their temperament, desires and aversions.

Avoid experimentation on laboratory animals.

Lack of expiration of the homeopathic medicine.

Homeopathy treats the patient and the disease in a totally individualized way. The same disease, in the same patient, but at a different time, will require a different treatment.
Healing is achieved through the activation of the body's defense mechanisms, which react appropriately thanks to the treatment.

Any substance existing in nature, whether of vegetable, animal or mineral origin, can be used as a homeopathic remedy.

For its effectiveness, a much more complete diagnosis is needed than those usually performed, which leads to a better cure.

Not only the physical health is taken into account, but also the emotional, family, work, environmental, genetic and cultural state, which leads to a complete clinical history of the real causes of the disease. Once these are known, the treatment is simpler and more accurate.

The medical specialty is eliminated and with it the current problem of the same patient being treated by different doctors, with different opinions.

The doctor-patient relationship is much more complete, since the psyche and the body are analyzed together.

Homeopathic medicine

The homeopathic medicine does not work by the amount of drug ingested, but by its dynamic effect that lasts more or less time according to the power of reaction or sensitivity of the organism and the degree of dynamization of the medicine, therefore, it does not accumulate, nor is it eliminated by urine, excrement, gas exchange, various secretions or skin, as it usually happens in allopathy. The elimination reactions that may cause diarrhea, sweating, various rashes, are not elimination of the drug, but rather toxins. The medication is given to the patient in subtle doses, so small that without causing pain or weakness are just enough to suspend the natural disease, which results that without causing discomfort, pain or weakness, the natural disease is extinguished.

Homeopathic preparations are obtained from products, substances, compositions from the plant, animal and mineral kingdoms. The strains of vegetable origin come from whole plants, leaves, branches, bark, roots, fruits, collected in their natural habitat. The use of dried or cultivated plants is exceptional, only when the wild plants required are in danger of extinction. Strains of animal origin come from whole animals, parts, organs or secretions of these. In strains of mineral origin, the raw material coincides with the base product, although they can also be products or mixtures obtained from the base substance.

These drugs can be consumed by infants and pregnant women. They do not cause dependence and are effective in the treatment of patients with a variety of disorders, both acute and chronic, acting at the cellular and molecular level by stimulating the reaction capacity, mobilizing the individual defense mechanisms.

When a homeopathic remedy is administered in a serious or chronic disorder, a homeopathic aggravation may occur. This is where the symptoms of the particular ailment worsen and it appears that the animal is getting worse. This relationship is due to changes in the body from the homeopathic remedy and is a sign that you have the correct remedy. A homeopathic reaction can last a couple of days or a week depending on the case being treated. An aggravation may be followed by an improvement. On the other hand, another remedy may be selected to continue.

The efficacy of homeopathic treatment

In homeopathy, the speed and effectiveness of a treatment depends, logically, as in allopathy, on a correct diagnosis and correct therapeutic indication.

If a patient is given an incorrect diagnosis, the medication will therefore not be effective. This does not mean, therefore, that homeopathy is useless. E.g.: If a patient who goes to a homeopathic physician with a liver problem is prescribed a medication primarily for circulatory problems, it will hardly be effective.

Homeopathy is not an alternative or complementary medicine, since, being a medical system studied, researched and applied for more than 200 years, it enjoys its own doctrine and widely proven. It is considered official medicine in many countries around the world, which even have exclusively homeopathic hospitals.

Diagnosis, prognosis and treatment are always subject to the criterion of psychophysical totality. This characteristic is, for the time being, one of the conditions for which the traditional medical criterion rejects it, but it is also one of the conditions for which the common people are interested in it. Without failing to recognize the great advances that the criterion of specialization brings to patients. Medications should be administered 30 minutes after feeding or 20 minutes before feeding.

Classification of homeopathic medicines

The best medicine in homeopathy is the constitutional medicine, which is the medicine of individual selection and prescription. Animals and humans treated with the constitutional medicine become less ill. Medicines obtained from secretions or pathological tissues Nosodes or biotherapeutics prepared by the homeopathic method of dilution and successive succussions described by Hahnemann have been used successfully.

Biotherapeutics are chemically undefined products (secretions, pathological or non-pathological excretions, certain products of microbial origin, allergens) that serve as raw materials for the preparation of their homeopathic use.

Biotherapeutics "Codees": are those obtained from serums, vaccines, toxins or anatoxins, registered in the French pharmacopoeia and prepared in a specialized laboratory. (Avina, Diphterotoxinum, Gonotoxinum, Tuberculinum).

Simple Biotherapeutics: They are elaborated from stock vaccines, constituted by microbial cultures, pure, lysed and attenuated under certain conditions. (Collibacillium, Ebertinum, Enterococcinum, Strectococcinum).

Complex biotherapeutics: They are defined by their mode of obtaining (secretions or pathological excretions) or by their mode of preparation. (Antracinum, Luesinum, Morbillinum, Pertissinum).

Biotherapeutics prepared from live microorganisms: Obtained from preparations with live microorganisms on the decimal scale, using 0.9% sodium chloride as diluent.

With this system, using an "isopathic" criterion (preventing in this case a disease with the same disease that produces it), it is possible to achieve immunity of variable duration according to
the dilution used and its frequency of repetition, for various infectious diseases (Diphtheria, Meningitis, Meningococcal, Measles).

The use of appropriate biotherapeutics in the acute phase of the infection will allow the rapid elimination of the infectious agent and its toxins, at the moment when the production of antibodies is just beginning, thus decreasing the time of the disease, the capacity to produce placebo effects of the remedy, of the patient and of the physician. However, the use of placebo does not have to be undignified and inadvisable and in many cases allows the administration of an active remedy and its consequence.

Homeopathic and allopathic Pharmacopoeia

They are official forms containing the preparations that can be dispensed by the pharmacist. The homeopathic medicine must always be prepared identically to the one used for the pathogenic experience, i.e., there can only be one preparation formula, although not all pharmacopoeias establish exactly the same rules for the preparations. The allopathic pharmacopoeia mostly contains a table of dosages of those drugs reported to be dangerous and toxic. The reason is that allopathic medicine bases the therapeutic action of its measurement on the amount of drug administered.

In homeopathy the most important thing is to put the patient in contact with the remedy. In theory, only one granule or globule would be enough to achieve this. However, a larger number is always prescribed to ensure that it is effective, but we must not forget that the homeopathic medicine acts at an exclusively qualitative level and therefore the amount of dose is not important.

Preparation of homeopathic medicines

The preparation of medicines involves knowledge of: Drugs, origin, collection, composition and of the operating manual of official preparations, mother tinctures and solutions.

Plant-derived products:

Whole plants, fresh or dried, or parts thereof.

Physiological (sarcodes), liquid or solid.

Alkaloids.

Glucose.

Resins.

Gomo-resins.

Mucilage.

Pathological (nosodes)

Animal by-products:

Whole animals, live, dead, or part of them fresh or dried.

Physiological: Secretions of healthy animals. Example: ostreic calcareous, etc. Pathological: Bacteria or their toxins, diseased organs or their secretions. Ex: tuberculin, syphilin, etc.

Organotherapy (hormones): Fresh or dried organ or its secretions. Examples: thyroid, thyroxine, ovary.

Autoisotherapy (autovaccine): Physiological or pathological product of a patient, to cure his own disease.

Natural products or products from the chemical-pharmaceutical industry.

Natural origin (purified or not). Example: metals and metalloids.

Industrial origin (natural or synthetic). E.g.: organic and inorganic salts, vitamins, hormones.

Exclusively homeopathic preparations.

Examples: Causticum, Mercurius solubilis.
One of the principles of homeopathy is the law of the minimum or infinitesimal dose. Hahnemman, who was also a chemist, determined with precision the operations to be carried out, highlighting a fundamental element: dynamization. It consists of applying after each dilution a precise number of agitations or suction. If the substance is diluted in solid excipients, this dynamization is carried out by trituration in a mortar.

The pharmaceutical forms used in homeopathy do not differ substantially from those already known in allopathic medicine. There are two therapeutic forms whose use can be considered specific to the homeopathic remedy: the tube of granules and the tube of globules. Their route of administration is sublingual.

Tube of granules: These are small spheres consisting of lactose and sucrose in a proportion of 15 % and 85 % with a mass of 50 mg. The tube contains 80 granules with a total weight of **49.**

Tube of globules or dose tube: These are spheres made of lactose and sucrose and their mass is 5 mg (10 times less than the granule), containing about 200 globules and weighing 1 g, it is also called dose tube because it takes the content only once, letting it be absorbed under the tongue.

Tablets: Lactose and sucrose with a mass of 100 mg.

Drops: Alcohol of 30 to 60 degrees is used. Also a mixture of glycerin, alcohol and

water.

Drinkable ampoules: These are ampoules of 1 or 2 mL with 15% alcohol.
Powders: Used for insoluble substances in dilutions up to 3 0C. The excipient is lactose.

Suppositories: The homeopathic dilution prepared in 30 proof alcohol is added to the excipient at the rate of 0.25 g for a 2 g suppository. The excipient is usually semi-synthetic glyceride with cocoa butter.

Ointments: Dilutions are incorporated in the excipient (vaseline or vasolanoline) in proportion of 4%.

Starting from a mother tincture, which is obtained by maceration of the substance in alcohol, the different dilutions are made by successive operations in the centesimal or decimal proportion. Normally the dilutions 5, 7, 9, 9, 15 and 30 are used, both decimal and centesimal, although in specific cases and by veterinary prescription these can vary up to 200 or even 1 000. The principle of the minimum dose is the one that has caused so much criticism of homeopathic medicine, since for some people it is difficult to understand how such a small amount of medicine can have any effect on the body. In this regard we can say the following: not all medicines are prescribed in infinitesimal doses, and those that are so prescribed, it is for their efficacy that both clinically and experimentally has been proven over the years.

High dynamizations are those we use for patients with a symptomatic totality in which mental symptoms predominate. Low dynamizations are used in acute cases, to treat local or physical symptoms, for example fever. Although it is hard to believe, the more diluted the remedy is, the more potent its action. We already know that beyond the dynamization 12, the number of Abogadro is exceeded, so there would be no more original substance and the preparation becomes 100% energy. Preparing a medicine requires a series of care and artisanal steps and only pharmacies specialized in the homeopathic technique can guarantee a 100% effective medicine. This is a detail that should be taken into account. To such an extent that it is one of the first points we consider in those cases in which the patient returns to the consultation with little or none of the expected result.

Vehicles and routes of administration of homeopathic medicines

The vehicle is very important because it becomes an integral part of the medicines. Not just any vehicle can be used, as homeopathic experimentation has been practiced with alcohol or triturations with milk sugar.

According to Hahnemman in some cases the healing power is in a latent state, it is necessary to awaken it; this activation or development by an almost destruction of the primitive matter and is practiced with the help of the vehicle lactose in trituration and alcohol in dynamization that receive the medicinal virtue of the substances exalted in their development and transmit it to the organism.

The most commonly used vehicles in homeopathy are: Distilled water, alcohol in different grades, glycerin, milk sugar, saccharin globules and lactose tablets.

The homeopathic medicine can be administered through the mucous membranes (tongue, mouth and stomach), upper respiratory tract (nose and pharynx) and lower respiratory tract, and the skin surface and the entire intact epidermis.

Preservation of homeopathic medicines

Homeopathic medicines need a minimum of care for their handling, normal temperature ranges, protection from sunlight, keeping away from substances that give off strong odors, perfumes, camphor, keeping the bottle tightly closed, not handling the medicine and not returning unused medicines to the bottle. As a general rule, as well as the orthodox ones, they should only be taken when they are necessary and left when they are no longer needed. The efficiency of the remedies depends on the similarity of the symptoms experienced with the remedy information.

Factors influencing the administration of homeopathic medicines

When administering a homeopathic remedy, a therapeutic act is synthesized in which important factors such as the patient, the disease and the physician have to be taken into account.

1.   Patient:

Age: In a young person or animal we can repeat the medication more frequently than in older people or animals.

Constitution: When weak, the dose will be smaller and the frequency of administration lower than in those organisms with a strong constitution.

Sensitivity: Whenever there is hypersensitivity it cannot be repeated often, small doses are given and it is better to start with low dynamizations.

2.   Disease:

Acute: One dose may be sufficient if the disease is not severe.

Chronic: More than one dose and dynamization is necessary for its cure. Functional: They are more tolerant of high dynamizations.

Structural: Treatment should be started at low dilutions and repeated with doses.

3. Physician:

It must have a method that allows integrating the variables that can be found, as well as facilitating the analysis of any event and, therefore, finding its solution, in addition to working with an administration method that makes it possible to ensure the exercise.

Let's take a closer look at all these aspects

Bases or principles

It is considered as a harmless therapy par excellence, it is extremely safe if correctly indicated. It has also been described as the therapeutic form that, based on the principle of similarity, uses the medicine in <u>Infinitesimal Doses</u> to cure; these are the two fundamental characteristics of Homeopathy. However, more strictly speaking, what truly defines and characterizes the homeopathic method is <u>Similarity</u>: without Similarity there is no Homeopathy. There are several therapeutics that use the "Weak Dose": trace elements, gemmotherapy. Homeopathy distinguishes itself from all of them and is characterized by the application of the principle of <u>Similitude</u> (Berthier, 1991).

<u>Principle of Similarity</u>: It consists of prescribing to a sick person or animal that medicine that when tested on a healthy individual has produced a symptomatic picture "similar" to the one presented by the sick person or animal. Hahnemann explains this principle in a clear and simple way: "The most effective medicine in each specific case will be similar to the one whose symptoms are similar to the disease to be treated" (Grosso, 1987).

<u>Infinitesimal doses</u>: Since its inception, the use of weak doses has aroused controversy and rejection by Classical Medicine. However, this peculiar administration of medicinal substances is not a product of a preconceived or intellectual approach. The updating of weak doses is, once again, the product of varied and repeated experiences, an observation drawn from practice. In this respect it is worth quoting Hahnemann's words: "It is not by virtue of a preconceived opinion, nor for love of singularity, that I decided in favor of weak doses. I have arrived at them by observation and they have shown me that many medicines act with more intensity to bring about a cure. Thus I have decreased them and as I have always observed the same effects, although to a lesser degree, I have gone down to the minimum doses" (Abecassis, 1985 and Berthier, 1991).

Substances that at their weighted doses are capable of provoking in healthy and sensitive individuals a certain symptomatological picture, are capable of making these same symptoms disappear in a patient who presents them if they are prescribed in small doses (Briones, 1990).

According to Jayasuriya (1988), the essence of Hahnermann's teaching is the similar remedy, simple drug, small dose, infrequent dose, non-interference with the vital reactions of the organism, initial aggravation (sometimes) and potentiation of the remedy. For this author himself, the basic rules of Homeopathy are:

- ❖ The law of similars.

- ❖ The law of evidence.

- ❖ The law of the sole remedy.

- ❖ The law of minimum doses and drug dynamization (potency) theory.

- ❖ The law of the direction of the cure.

- ❖ The law of the doctrine of the Miasmas.

The law of similars

This law forms the key to homeopathic practice. The bases that allowed Hahnemann to formulate this law were the following:

a) That any symptom complex or syndrome is not the disease as such, but the defense action mechanism mobilized by the body in contact with an influence is what causes the disease, being this a specific stress such as a bacterium or virus, or a non-specific stress such as climatic changes, environmental pollution, emotional or mental disturbances, among others.

b) That the symptoms do not constitute the disease, but that the reactions of the organism under stress are the means by which the organism attempts against its lost physiological balance (homeostasis).

An organized system in equilibrium responds to any particular disturbance force at the optimum time.

c) That, in order to help the organism restore its order, the physician should assist and reinforce these reactions rather than suppress them. The correct homeopathic remedy is chosen by assuming that the patient is extremely receptive to that particular remedy and only that specific remedy, which is capable of producing his symptomatology.

"Simila Similibus Curantur" can be explained as the same substance capable of producing the specific symptoms in a healthy individual; it can cure a patient of a disease by producing identical or similar symptoms.

d) Suppression of symptoms (known as contrapathy or antipathy) is one of the major dangers of allopathic medicine. The contraria contraris paradigm is used in Oriental medicine to oppose the symptoms of disease.

The Law of Evidence

Hahnemann experimented on groups of healthy human volunteers, including himself, by orally taking medicinal plants, minerals and animal substances. He found that when active medicinal materials are ingested by humans in sufficient quantity, they produce a pattern of symptoms, which initiate a natural disease, either acute or chronic.

The Law of the Single Remedy

The one who wishes to perform an ultimate cure on the patient must prescribe one and only one specific remedy that has produced in his tests, the greatest similarity to the complex of symptoms present in a patient. Any other remedy will have no real curative effect.
The single remedy is all that is needed, presenting the advantage that when a remedy is administered its action can be evaluated. However, if a group of remedies are administered, it is not possible to evaluate or know which one cured, or in what proportion.

This is known as individualization. However, there are many remedies that have a broad spectrum of action, and these are used when the disease exhibits diverse and sometimes vague symptomatology. Other groups of patients show characteristics in common, using in these cases remedies known as constitutional.

The Law of Minimum Dose (homeopathic dose)

When homeopathy found the relevant individual remedy, the specific allergen to which an allergic person was sensitive was discovered.

It is understood by this that in homeopathy the homeopath has to prescribe a very small dose, in order not to cause an enormous aggravation of the patient's symptomatology.

This law is compatible with the Arnolt-Schultz Law, which states that small doses stimulate, medium doses paralyze and large doses kill. According to this law, the action of small and very large doses of the same substance of living matter is opposite.

After the initial micro dose has acted on the patient, it will bring a healing response through a sequence of internal cascading events, such as the reinforcement of defense mechanisms, reestablishing the vital balance with the organism.

In this way, the remedy acts as a catalytic agent and usually does not need to be repeated frequently. In addition, the pharmaceutical cost of homeopathic treatment is lower. Homeopathy is safe, simple, effective, non-invasive and an economical mode of therapy. Its iatrogenic effects are minimal. The initial aggravation of the patient's symptoms is followed by a total improvement which, together with the observation of the Law of Cure, is a confirmation that an ultimate repair of health has taken place and not a suppression.

Curation Management Act
The reestablishment of the internal order and the consequent return to health of the sick individual was observed to follow a predictable pattern. In the progressive march of symptoms as the cure occurs, it is noted that the main symptomatology moves from the most vital, to the less vital functional centers within the organism. In other words, from the vital organs to the skin, from the mental to the emotional and finally to the physical. In the healing process, the rapid reappearance of old symptoms is also noted as a residue of the previous suppressed disease, making its way to the periphery to be eliminated by the homeopathically reinforced defense.

By giving the true simillium, the symptoms are cured according to Hering's laws:

1. Pain improvement takes place from top to bottom.

2. The improvement of diseases occurs from the inside out.

3. The symptoms of a disease disappear in the same order in which they appeared, the most important or vital organs being relieved first, then the less important ones, and the mucous membranes and skin last.

4. Kent adds this fourth aspect: As the last appeared symptoms of the last disease disappear, the symptoms of old suppressed diseases reappear and disappear as soon as they appear.

As in all holistic and natural healing systems, the process involves an initial aggravation of the symptom as a defense mechanism. In a successful homeopathic treatment the initial elimination phase with the average presentation of symptoms is quickly followed by an improvement of all symptoms and return to normal health. The cure is considered complete when there is a total reestablishment of normal vital functions, expressed as optimal function of the mental, emotional and physical spheres of life.

The Doctrine of the Miasmas

This was Hahnemann's hypothesis to explain many disorders, which seemed to be based on hereditary-familial treatises. He classified them as Psora, Psychosis and Syphilis. This shows his ingenuity in talking about genetics and transmissible disorders.
at a time before Mendel, when little was understood on this subject, which led to the admission that each disease was unique and individual, but can occur in common.

At present, for Guajardo (1994), the principles of homeopathic medicine are eight:

❖ Pathogenesis.

❖ Activated polar solvents (Physicochemistry of homeopathic dynamo-dilution).

❖ Principle of similarity

❖ Pathological individuality

❖ Medicinal individuality

❖ Healing Bio-cybernetics

❖ Body Bio-energy

❖ Multifactorial genetic diseases (miasmatic predisposition)
A few years later, Fernandez (1998), cites the homeopathic principles as follows:

❖ Principle of similarity: states that a remedy cures a disease when it is capable of producing in a healthy person the same symptoms as those of the sick person.

❖ Principle of infinitesimal dosage: refers to the preparation of the homeopathic remedy, based on a process of successive dilutions alternating with suction.

❖ Principle of individuality and totality: there are no diseases but sick people. Each individual manifests the disease in a characteristic way and taking the globality of the symptoms presented by the patient (mental, general, local, modalities) it is determined which is the remedy that will cure the patient.

The disease

Article 6 of the Organon postulates a homeopathic concept of disease which refers to the fact that changes in the health of the body and mind can be perceived by means of the senses, that is, they are felt by the patient himself, are observed by those around him and are noticed by the physician; this set of perceptible symptoms forms the true and unique picture of the disease (Hahnemann, 1999). It is the patient as a whole who requires the physician's assistance and not just a liver disorder, a cardiac lesion or laryngitis.
Despite its basically symptomatological character, homeopathy does not neglect in any case the etiology or the causes that trigger disorders. Homeopathy in no case opposes or excludes surgery, supportive therapies and hygiene rules (Briones, 1996).

In chronic diseases with frequent relapses, immediate similarity is not enough to cure the patient; it is necessary to go further and attack the predisposing factors that Hahnemann called chronic Miasmas (Briones, 1996):

Psora miasma is the set of pathologies related to immunosuppression, autoimmune phenomena and allergy. The basics of this miasma would be the cyclical appearance of acute phenomena, the predominance of eruptive and pruritic skin affections, articular affections and intestinal disorders, the convalescence of very long acute diseases and the lack of response to homeopathic medicine, even if it is the most indicated.

Syphilis is interpreted as the pathological tendency with great affinity with the cardiovascular, bone and nervous system. This miasma is dominated by ulcerations, chronic purulent lesions and tissue sclerosis. The diseases are often irreversible.

Sycosis can be considered as congenital, corresponding to the hydrogenoid type with adiposity of the lower body and tendency to edema; or acquired, mainly due to the abuse of corticosteroids, anti-inflammatory drugs or antibiotics that have determined an immune deficiency with low reactivity.

Tuberculinism would be treated as a situation that affects mainly young individuals, with inability to adapt to the environment and extreme sensitivity to cold and drafts. It is characteristic the tendency to suffer respiratory problems, thinness with good appetite, tendency to headaches, diarrhea and otalgias and some types of allergy.

Undoubtedly one of the problems facing the homeopath today is the need to discern whether he/she is dealing with a real acute disease or with the acute manifestation of a chronic disease.

Kent summarizes: You cannot say that an individual is sick because he has a white tumor on his knee, but that he has a white tumor on his knee because he is sick.

In an acute patient, three clinical aspects clearly predominate: pain, fever and alterations in the functioning of an organ or group of organs.

Hahnemann (1999), refers in the reprinted edition of the Organon of Medicine, that when an organism falls ill, it is only the immaterial and active vital force by itself and present in all parts of the organism, which suffers of course the deviation that determines the dynamic influence of the morbid agent hostile to life. The homoeopathic method is employed to activate this vital force since it has the power and the tendency to produce an artificial morbid state similar to the pathological case in question.

The following examples are a sample of the above:

• The old reaper never drinks cold water when the burning sun and the fatigue of work have given him a burning fever; on the contrary, he drinks a little exciting liquor, a shot of aguardiente.

• The cook who has just burned his hand, presents it to the fire, at a certain distance, without paying attention to the increase of pain that results at first, because by acting in this way and in a short time he succeeds in perfectly curing the burn and making the slightest pain disappear.

• Limbs that have just frozen are rubbed with snow.

Mechanisms of action

Homeopathy is a reactive therapy, whose medicines induce self-healing mechanisms and are immuno-modulators. Healing can only take place by reaction of the vital force against the correct medicine taken (Briones, 1996; De Medio, 1997; I.B.E.H.E, 1997; Silva, 1998 and Paschero, 1999).
Homeopathy works effectively with reversible disorders, due to its biophysical basis and is based on stimulating the bioenergetic capacity of each living organism so that it fights and resolves the irregularity presented (Taubin, 1959; Dyson, 1971 and Periódico Granma, 1997). The remedy does not cure by substance but by its energetic capacity to excite a natural reactive complex (Paschero, 1999).

The homeopathic medicine does not work by the amount of drug ingested, but by its dynamic effect that lasts more or less time according to the power of reaction or sensitivity of the organism and the degree of dynamization of the medicine, therefore, it does not accumulate, nor is it eliminated through urine, excrement, gas exchange, various secretions or through the skin, as it usually happens in allopathy. The elimination reactions that may cause diarrhea, sweating, various rashes, are not elimination of the drug, but rather toxins (Cummings, 1991).

The problem in terms of homeopathic dosage then lies in the minimum amount of medicine that is capable of producing the desired effect: contrary to the method followed by the allopathic school, whose criterion is always to use the highest dose, according to the tolerance of the patient to achieve its objective (Speight, 1995).

The mechanism of action of homeoprophylaxis can be explained homeopathically in terms of predisposition or sensitivity, something called in homeopathy as idiosyncrasy (Golden, 1999).

The mechanism of action of homeopathic medicines is still an enigma on the way to be clarified in this 21st century; here are some of the hypotheses and discoveries of the late 20th century (Celorio, 1999).

In relation to the solvent configuration:

LIQUID CRYSTALS: there were ordered, disordered or amorphous crystals and it was thought that liquids had no structure, but in the 80's liquid crystals or quasi-crystals emerged as an intermediate stage (mesomorphic) of matter, ordered systems, but not periodic, which could describe a large number of phenomena not previously accessible. Crystals have demonstrated the ability to memorize. Their growth is wave-like in nature, which could explain the oscillatory tendency of homeopathic drugs.

In a solution, each solute crystal is surrounded by several water molecules (up to 15,000 per protein molecule), and each water layer vibrates at a specific frequency determined by the solute. By dynamizing a drug, the succussion forms new liquid crystals, and although they no longer contain molecules of the solute, they maintain the same structural and energetic pattern.

The liquid crystal has an electric dipole that generates a strong electromagnetic field and attracts neighboring particles that make it grow. As they fragment, they continue to grow and successive succussions and dilutions result in their growth and multiplication.

Salas Cuevas, a Mexican biophysicist, suggested in 1989 that the liquid crystals of the solvent remain as swarms of particles in a mesomorphic state, depending on the degree of association, depending on the dimensions of the original solute type.

In relation to the way of conserving and transmitting the information:

DIPOLE EFFECT: the electromagnetic field of a molecule suspended in water generates a permanent polarization of water dipoles that enables it to transmit radiant fields, therefore, there is a permanent electric polarization around an electrically polarized impurity (solute). The coherent interaction between the electric dipoles of water and the electromagnetic field generates ordered structures, the water becomes coherent. During succussion, water close to the molecule can act as a transmission agent and generate a permanent polarization in thousands of molecules around it.

MEMORY OF WATER: Cyril Smith discovered that water is able to memorize the electrical resonance it has received in tests with patients who reacted with allergy when in contact with water irradiated at the corresponding allergen frequency. The effect was reproduced even with sealed glass containers and at some distance from the allergic subject.

All living cells act as emitters or receivers of electromagnetic radiation, because cell organelles, such as mitochondria, seem to have the characteristic of adapted oscillating electronic circuits. Health would be given by a harmonious resonance between its organelles and disease as an imbalance.

produced either by an alteration of the electrical properties of the cell or by being subjected to excessive radiation from an external source. Chromosomes are the most important cellular oscillators.

Nuclear magnetic resonance has shown that there is subatomic activity in homeopathic remedies compared to placebos, which have none. In England, several studies have been done and it points out that homeopathy has already been proven. Through 4.5 years of extensive clinical research, it was shown that a homeopathic treatment for hay fever was much more powerful than a placebo. The surprising results were published in the medical journal, Lancet in 1986 (Solorzano, 2003).

Advantages

According to Fernandez (1998), Homeopathy has advantages over conventional medicine:

❖ Individualization of treatment in view of symptoms.

❖ Absence of drug toxicity, avoiding the accumulation of toxic residues in slaughter animals and their production.

❖ Application of this therapeutic in the new trends of animal production aimed at obtaining ecological productions.

❖ Absence of side effects.

❖ Ease of administration.

❖ It helps to improve the knowledge about our animal, its temperament, its desires and aversions.

❖ Lack of expiration of the homeopathic medicine.

Agustí (1998), for his part, points out as advantages:

❖ Homeopathy treats the patient and the disease in a totally individualized way. The same disease, in the same patient, but at a different time, will require a different treatment.

❖ Healing is achieved through the activation of the body's defense mechanisms, which react appropriately thanks to the treatment.

❖ There is no danger of toxicity, even in prolonged treatments.

❖ Any substance existing in nature, whether of vegetable, animal or mineral origin, can be used as a homeopathic remedy.

❖ For its effectiveness, a much more complete diagnosis is needed than those usually performed, which leads to a better cure.

❖ Not only the physical health is taken into account, but also the emotional, family, work, environmental, genetic and cultural state, which leads to a complete clinical history of the real causes of the disease. Once these are known, the treatment is simpler and more accurate.

❖ The medical specialty is eliminated and with it the current problem of the same patient being treated by different doctors, with different opinions.

❖ The doctor-patient relationship is much more complete, since the psyche and the body are analyzed together.

Notions of homeopathic pharmacology

This is the most controversial point for its understanding, and also for its acceptance by physicians of other specialties, since the medicine that comes from natural sources (vegetable, animal or mineral), or from pathological products (pus, flows, bacteria, stones, etc.), must meet 2 important requirements, which are: the repeated dilutions to which it is subjected reaching concentrations below 10, which exceeds Avogadro's number and, therefore, there is no quantifiable molecule, and the dimanization, which are violent agitations that are printed to the medicine. Advances in physics, mathematics, bio-cybernetics, biochemistry and other sciences have not yet covered all the doubts on this subject, but the reality is one: drugs cure, alleviate or modify the disease (Riverón, 1997).

In spite of the fact that in 1839 the use of homeopathic medicine was known in Cuba, and that it reached an excellent development, its use was almost abandoned in the second half of the 19th century for several reasons; however, it has taken off in recent years in the field of human and veterinary medicine. As a contribution to the development of this discipline in Cuba, an inventory of vegetable species used in the preparation of homeopathic medicines, native or exotic that are cultivable in the island, is offered. It presents 96 species, grouped in 91 genera of 47 families. All the species included have references of medicinal uses in allopathic medicine and 20 of them have some reference of toxicity (Fuentes, 1996).

The strains of vegetable origin come from whole plants, leaves, branches, bark, roots, fruits, collected in their natural habitat. The use of dried or cultivated plants is exceptional, only when the wild plants required are in danger of extinction. The strains of animal origin come from whole animals, parts, organs or secretions of these. In strains of mineral origin, the raw material coincides with the base product, although they can also be products or mixtures obtained from the base substance (Fernández, 1998).

This author posits that drug preparation involves knowledge of:

1. Drugs, origin, collection, composition.

2. Operating manual of official preparations, mother tinctures, solutions.

Origin of medicines.

<u>Plant kingdom:</u>

❖ Products derived from plants: Whole plants or parts thereof, fresh or dried.

Physiological (sarcodes), liquid or solid.

-       Alkaloids.

-       Glucose.

-       Resins.

-       Gomo-resins.

-       Mucilage.

Pathological (nosodes)

From them, the MOTHER DYE (TM) is obtained.

The T.M. has an expiration date of 5 years.

<u>MOTHER TINCTURE</u> (1/10):

1 Collection

2.   - Selection

3.   - Moisture determination

4.   - Alcoholic maceration (70° alcohol is used)

5.   - Decanting

6.   - Expression

7.   - Mixing

8.   - Rest

9.   - Filtration

10.   - Conservation

<u>Animal kingdom:</u>

❖ Products derived from animals: Whole animals, live, dead, or part of them fresh or dried.

-        Physiological (sarcodes): Secretions of healthy animals. Example: calcareous, buffalo, cuttlefish, etc.

-        Pathological (nosodes): Bacteria or their toxins, diseased organs or their secretions. Example: tuberculin, syphilin, etc.
-        Organotherapy (hormones): Fresh or dried organ or its secretions. Example: thyroid, thyroxine, ovary, etc.

-        Autoisotherapy (autovaccine): Physiological or pathological product of a patient, to cure his own disease.

<u>Mineral kingdom:</u>

❖ Natural products or products from the chemical-pharmaceutical industry.

-        Natural origin (purified or not). Example: metals and metalloids.
-        Industrial origin (natural or synthetic). Example: inorganic and organic salts, vitamins, hormones.

❖ Exclusively homeopathic preparations.

Example: Heparsulfur, Causticum, Mercurius solubilis.

Dilutions and dynamizations

As mentioned above, one of the principles of homeopathy is the law of the minimum or infinitesimal dose. Hahnemman, who was also a chemist, determined with precision the operations to be carried out, highlighting a fundamental element: dynamization. It consists of applying after each dilution a precise number of agitations or suction. If the substance is diluted in solid excipients, this dynamization is carried out by trituration in a mortar.

Starting from the mother tincture, which is obtained by maceration of the substance in alcohol, the different dilutions are made by successive operations in the centesimal or decimal proportion. Normally the dilutions 5, 7, 9, 9, 15 and 30 are used, both decimal and centesimal, although in specific cases and by veterinary prescription these can vary up to 200 or even 1 000 (Fernandez, 1998).

The principle of the minimum dose is the one that has provoked so much criticism of homeopathic medicine, since for some people it is difficult to understand how such a small amount of medicine can have any effect on the organism. In this regard we can say the following: not all medicines are prescribed in infinitesimal doses, and those that are so prescribed, it is for their efficacy that both clinically and experimentally has been proven over the years (Flores and Flores, 1999).

To restore the lost balance of the organism there are 2 solutions:

1. Forces are used to combat the undesirable invader and the annoying symptoms it causes (this is one of the principles of allopathy: Antibiotics, Antidepressants, Antispasmodics, etc.).

2. Natural defenses are stimulated to make them more effective. This is the mechanism of Homeopathy (Anonymous, 2000).

High dynamodilutions are used for patients with a symptomatic totality in which mental symptoms predominate. Low dynamodilutions are used in acute cases, to treat local or physical symptoms, e.g. fever. The more diluted the remedy is, the more potent the action. And we know that beyond the dynamodilution 12, Avogadro's number is exceeded so there would be no more original substance becoming the preparation 100% energy. Preparing a medicine requires a series of care and artisanal steps and only pharmacies specialized in the homeopathic technique can guarantee a 100% effective medicine. This is a detail that should be taken into account, to such an extent that it is one of the first points that we consider in those cases in which the patient returns to the consultation with little or none of the expected result (Pereira, **2000**).

Guillén (1994) states that the pharmaceutical forms used in homeopathy do not differ substantially from those already known in allopathic medicine. There are two forms whose use can be considered specific to the homeopathic remedy: the tube of granules and the tube of globules. Their route of administration is sublingual.

Pharmaceutical forms

1. Tube of granules: they are small spheres consisting of lactose and sucrose in a proportion of 15 % and 85 % with a mass of 50 mg. The tube contains 80 granules with a total weight of 4 g.

2.   Tube of globules or dose tube: they are also spheres made up of lactose and sucrose and their mass is 5 mg (10 times less than the granule), containing about 200 globules and weighing 1 g. It is also called dose tube because it takes the content only once, leaving it to be absorbed under the tongue.

3. Tablets: they are made of lactose and sucrose with a mass of 100 mg.

4. Drops: alcohol from 30 to 60 degrees is used. In addition, a mixture of

glycerin, alcohol and water.

5. Drinkable ampoules: 1 or 2 ml_ ampoules with 15% alcohol.

6. Powders: used for insoluble substances in dilutions up to 3 C. The excipient is lactose.

7. Suppositories: the homeopathic dilution prepared in alcohol 30 v/v is added to the excipient due to 0.25 g for a 2 g suppository. The excipient is usually semi-synthetic glyceride with cocoa butter.

8. Ointments: dilutions are incorporated in the excipient (vaseline or vasolanoline) in proportion of 4%.

Vehicles

The vehicle is very important because it becomes an integral part of the medicines. Not just any vehicle can be used, since homeopathic experimentation has been practiced with alcohol or triturations with milk sugar (Suarez, 1989).

According to Hahnemman in some cases the healing power is in a latent state, it is necessary to awaken it; this activation or development by an almost destruction of the primitive matter is practiced with the help of the vehicle lactose in trituration and alcohol in dynamization that receive the medicinal virtue of the substances exalted in their development and transmit it to the organism (Martinez, 1990).

The most commonly used vehicles in Homeopathy are:

Distilled water.

Alcohol in different degrees.

Glycerin.

Milk sugar.

Saccharin globules.

Lactose tablets.

Pharmacopoeia

Pharmacopoeias are official forms containing the preparations that can be dispensed by the pharmacist. The homeopathic medicine must always be prepared identically to the one used for the pathogenic experience, i.e., there can only be one preparation formula, although not all pharmacopoeias establish exactly the same rules for the preparations (Barros, 1992).

In Homeopathy the most important thing is to put the patient in contact with the remedy. In theory, only one granule or globule would be enough to achieve this. However, a larger number is always prescribed to ensure that it is effective, but we must not forget that the homeopathic medicine acts at an exclusively qualitative level and therefore the amount of dose is not important (Schwabe, 1995).

The dosage will depend on the toxic level of the disease, i.e., its acute or chronic nature (Almunia et al., 1998).

Most commonly used dilutions.

- Centecimal (C) 1/100.

- Decimal (X, D) 1/10.

Low doses - TM up to 6 CH.

They act on the organs and their action is short.

Medium doses - 6 CH up to 30 CH.

They act on anatomical regions or systems with a medium effect.

High doses - 200 CH - 1000 CH and higher.
They act on the mental sphere, the nervous system and the total economy with prolonged effects (one dose every 15 days or more).

The dilution carried out according to the Hahnemannian method is performed by successive operations of repartition of the source in a vehicle either to 1/100 (centecimal) or to 1/10 (decimal).

The number of manipulations establishes the level of dilution. Dilution leads to obtaining liquid preparations called "dilutions" or solid preparations called "triturations" (Abecassis et al., 1984). To name these preparations, we use the following abbreviations:

Decimal dilutions or triturations: D or X.

Centecimal dilutions or triturations: C.

In any of the cases, depending on the pharmaceutical method used, the letters H, F or K will appear after the letter D, X or C, meaning:

H- by the Hahnemannian method (manual).

F- continuous fluxing (mechanical).

K- by Korsakov's method (mechanical).

Preservation of homeopathic medicines

According to Martínez (1990), homeopathic medicines require a minimum of care in handling, normal temperature ranges, protection from sunlight, keeping away from substances that give off strong odors, perfumes, camphor, keeping the bottle tightly closed, not handling the medicine and not returning unused medicines to the bottle.

Homeopathic medicines, as a general rule, like orthodox medicines, should only be taken when they are needed and discontinued when they are no longer needed.

They should be administered 30 minutes after feeding or 20 minutes before feeding.
They should be stored in a cool, dark place, away from food and other strong-smelling products, making sure that the lid is not damaged (Lockie and Geldir, 1995).

The conservation of the therapeutic effect is generally indefinite, and requires a series of indispensable precautions of preparation, adequate storage, careful handling and avoidance of contamination. In the Manual of Technical Standards of Homeopathic Pharmacy (1997), they refer to the causes that attribute or impede the conservation:

♦ Fermentation (happens to those with an alcoholic content of less than 60 degrees).

♦ Evaporation (the preparation becomes aqueous, does not lose its action, but cannot be used for embedding globules, tablets and slips) It would be more critical in very low dilutions.

♦ Moisture (between the lid and the mouth of the bottle, may promote fungal growth).

♦ Cork lid (with continuous use in the same bottle, it may alter the dilution).

♦ Heat (safest method to destroy a dynamization, 40 degrees and above).

♦ Magnetic fields (avoid approaching radio and TV speakers, or other media that transmit this energy).

♦ Aromas (both pleasant [perfumes or others] and unpleasant)

♦ Light (avoid direct or indirect sunlight and all types of light for prolonged exposures).

♦ Do not change medication from the original bottle.

♦ Do not touch tablets with your hands or the mouth of the bottle.

Homeopathy, possible uses in cases of disaster occurrence

In today's world, the practice of natural medicines is becoming more and more popular. This is due to their proven efficacy and innocuousness. Homeopathy is one of them and is defined as the medicine that deals with the study, diagnosis and treatment of the sick terrain (human or animal), according to the Law of Similarity. Its creator was the German Samuel Hahnemann, a German scholar who was born in the city of Meissen on April 10, 1755 and died in Paris on July 2, 1843. He initiated a new current in world medical thought where man and animal constitute a biology integrally related and in constant interchange in the environment.

It began to be practiced on humans and was later introduced in veterinary medicine, achieving encouraging results in all animal species that have been the object of research.

This medical system has achieved great prestige during the years that have elapsed since its emergence. In spite of this, there has been no lack of detractors who have harshly attacked it in an attempt to diminish its importance. However, homeopathy has been gaining followers and its practice has spread worldwide, with its principles coming to life more and more through clinical practice and experimentation.

It seems to be more than a coincidence that this gentle and safe therapeutic modality, without effects or contradictions, has allowed those who practice it to achieve longer than normal life spans, as is also the case for most of their patients, a fact that is confirmed by the death certificates of homeopathic physicians around the world, since homeopathy knows no borders.

It is a medical discipline whose primary emphasis is on therapy. It is a low-cost system that employs exclusively non-toxic drugs. It can be used to treat both acute and chronic cases, but its magnificent contribution lies in its successful treatment of chronic diseases, which have become difficult to manage by orthodox methods. It takes the sick individual and treats his disturbances in the physical, emotional and mental planes at the same time; managing to restore the lost balance of the sick individual at all three levels, through the stimulation and reinforcement of his defense mechanism (autoimmune system, reticuloendothelial system, hormonal system, sympathetic-parasympathetic system and the psychological mechanism that responds to stress). In short, this type of medicine is a reactive therapy, whose drugs induce self-healing mechanisms and are immuno-modulators.

Repertorization

A repertorization is an index of symptoms corresponding to homeopathic remedies that are systematically renewed. It can be stored alphabetically or in schematic order in the definitive principles of the guide, for easy reference.

It is a table or compendium of the symptomatology of the provings, where the content is arranged for easy reference, since no human mind is capable of memorizing all the Homeopathic Materia Medica.

A repertory is not a medical subject. In a repertory there is a separation of symptoms by analysis for the purpose of classification and for a readable reference. In the materia medica, the synthesis of the drug, the effects of its unit and its relationships are described in depth. Not all symptoms are of equal value. The mental ones (mood, mania, delirium, etc.) are those that occupy the first place, particularly when they mark in the person a notable change in his character, or mode of being, of his state of health. In second place, although of almost equal importance to the mental ones, are the general symptoms; these refer to how the whole organism reacts to the disease, to temperature, to food, to a certain position or posture, desire (cravings) or aversions. The local or particular symptoms, which are also common to several persons affected by the same disease, are of lesser importance for the selection of the medicine: pain, cough, fever, inflammation, appearance of the tongue, etc. The remedy should also cover these symptoms, but they should never be taken solely as a guide for the indication.

Homeopathic medicines that can be used in different diseases

Homeopathic medicines can be used in different ailments (prophylactic and therapeutic). They are effective in the treatment of acute or chronic conditions, according to the system or apparatus affected. The following is a brief description of some of the possible uses of homeopathic drugs.

For the treatment of gastroenteritis or diarrheal syndrome

Lachesis to dynamodilution 30 CH 10 drops (0.3 mL), 2 times a day orally. In cases with predominant symptoms such as: prostrations, greenish-yellow, frothy, mucous, bloody, hot and foul-smelling stools, as well as thick and serous nasal secretion.

Pulsatilla nigricans to the power of 200 CH 10 drops, 1 time a day orally. In cases of observed: prostrations, greenish-yellow, mucous and foul-smelling stools, neck stiffness and thick and serous nasal secretion.

Calcarea carbonicum at 30 CH 10 drops, 2 times a day orally, when symptoms predominate such as: prostrations, frothy and fetid stools, neck stiffness and thick and serous nasal secretion.

Sulphur at 30 CH potency 10 drops twice a day orally. When symptoms such as: prostrations, greenish-yellow, frothy, mucous and foul-smelling stools, neck stiffness, thick and serous nasal secretion and dryness of the ocular mucosa are evidenced.

Arsenicum album to dynamodilution 30 CH 10 drops (0.3 ml_), 2 times a day orally. When there are symptoms such as: Emaciation, frequent defecation, bloody and black stools.

Phosphorum a la 30 CH 10 drops (0.3 ml_), 2 times a day orally. When there is predominance: Emaciation, frequent defecation, bloody stools and continuous thirst.

Medications that may be indicated in hepatic conditions:

In acute or crisis cases due to biliary lithiasis they can be used.

Belladonna a la 30 CH 10 drops (0.3 ml_), 2 times a day orally. When symptoms such as: pain with violent onset and end, hypersensitivity to contact and movement, fever and headache.

Colocyntis: When the symptoms present correspond to visceral spasms.

Ricinus: It can be indicated in case of pain in the waist accompanied by diarrhea, while Bryonia in stabbing pain in the right hypochondrium produced or aggravated by movement, pressure, fever with intense thirst; also when there is bitter taste, tart tongue and dry mouth.
In chronic cases Berberis where gallstone colic is present, with jaundice and stabbing pain radiating to the left shoulder or abdomen.

Lycopodium: It is indicated in biliary lithiasis due to cholesterol and renal lithiasis due to urate, as well as in the presence of digestive symptoms such as pain in the right hypochondrium when lying on that side.

In patients suffering from hepatitis, a wide range of drugs can be administered such as: Apis, Bryonia, Arsenicum, Mercurios, China, Arsenicum, Lycopodium and Nux vomica.

Arsenicum: It should be applied when there is alternating agitation and prostration, asthenia, anxiety, congestive headaches, vomiting, burning diarrhea, pain, heat, thirst. Painful liver, tendency to anemia, pruritus and nocturnal heat. It can also be administered in cases of liver cirrhosis.

For the treatment of pneumonias and respiratory syndrome.

Pulsatilla at the potency of 30 CH 10drops (0.3 mL), 2 times a day orally. When symptoms such as: coryza, soft, yellowish or even green discharge, weakness and immunosuppression are observed.

Ipecac in 30 CH potency 10 drops (0.3 mL), 2 times a day orally.When symptoms such as: Expectoration, cough with sialorrhea and tongue not saburral.

Mercurius solubilis to the dynamo dilution of 30 CH 10drops (0.3 mL), 2 times a day orally. When symptoms such as: right bronchopneumopathy, purulent rhinorrhea and mercurial mouth are evidenced".

Hepar sulfur to the potency of 30 CH 10 drops (0.3 mL), 2 times a day orally. When symptoms such as: barking cough, hoarse, croup (laryngeal croup), after sudden cooling.

Euphrasia 30 CH 10 drops (0.3 mL) twice a day orally. When symptoms such as: coryza and mild rhinitis and conjunctivitis, keratoconjunctivitis with or without respiratory processes predominate.

Bryonia to the dynamodilution of 30 CH 10 drops (0.3 mL), 2 times a day orally. When symptoms that may occur: Those of respiratory syndrome of infectious origin, acute, dry cough of insidious onset and strong dyspnea or great respiratory distress.

Phosphorus a la 30 CH 10 drops (0.3 mL) 2 times a day orally When symptoms predominate as: Those of respiratory syndrome with hemorrhagic manifestations and right heart failure and pulmonary hypertension.

Belladonna 30 CH 10 drops (0.3 mL) twice a day orally. When symptoms predominate such as: Respiratory syndrome with cough and fever manifestations, head congestion and hyperesthesia.

Oscilococcinum (Anas barbarie) 13 CH and 204 CH. It can be used in offspring of any animal species or infants, 0.3 mL of the drug will be applied orally in single or repeated doses, up to three consecutive days.

Echinaceas at 7 CH and 30CH potency. It can be used in offspring of any species and infants, to which 0.3 mL of the drug will be applied orally in single or repeated doses for up to three consecutive days.

Cantharis compound to the dynamodilution 30 CH at the rate of 5 drops, every 6 hours until improvement, can be indicated in acute or chronic cystitis of various origins. Difficulty urinating, painful urination. In cases of gonorrhea and urethritis. Post antibiotic therapy in cases of urethral and bladder sepsis.

Sepia compuesta presents beneficial effects when indicated 5 drops sublingually, every 6-8 hours in gynecological disorders (infectious or non-infectious uterine inflammations, pyometra, dysmenorrhea, moniliasis and vaginal discharge.

Sebal compound can be administered 5 drops sublingually, every 6-8 hours until the patient improves.

In the prophylaxis and therapy of nervous disorders, homeopathic drugs are often indicated for anti-anxiety and antidepressant purposes:

Medications used in anxiety.

Aconitum:

Anxiety of paroxysmal presentation, intense, with a feeling of imminent death.

-With paresthesias, prechordalgia and palpitations.at midnight Chamomilla:

Choleric, quarrelsome character.

Hyperaesthesia to pain

Anger disorders (anxiety, abdominal pains)

Gelsemium:

Tremors, objective or subjective.

Vasomotor and sympathetic syndrome.

-Paresthesias.

Ignatia:

-Changing mood.

Sensitive to setbacks and distraction.

Dotted and erratic pains Antidepressant drugs.

Graphites:

-Sadness.

-Anguish with apprehension and indecision.

-Obesity.

Skin pathology (moist eczema, warts, keloids), digestive (dyspepsia, constipation), genital and sexual.

Kalium phosphoricum:

Depressed, very fatigued, adynamic. From great grief, very irritable, impatient, without memory.

Headaches.

Arsenicum album:

Intense fatigue with physical and mental agitation, anxiety.

Pessimistic, feels incurable. Meticulous, scrupulous.

For the treatment of conjunctivitis.

A homeopathic complex (EPA) against hemorrhagic conjunctivitis, consisting of Euphracia, Phosphorus and Apis, was successfully used in western Cuba during natural disasters (hurricanes).

For the treatment of dengue fever. Pharmacies in Rio de Janeiro, Brazil market a homeopathic remedy of natural origin to combat the symptoms of dengue fever. The homeopathic compound is based on a substance extracted from rattlesnake venom (Crotalus Horridus, Phosphorus, Eupatorium perf). The so-called Proden, developed and patented by Laboratorio Homeopático Almeida Prado, facilitates the recovery of patients who contract the disease and helps to prevent the disease. "The pill does not cause side effects and significantly reduces the recovery time of patients." Because it is a natural product, it apparently does not cause side effects. The drug was developed after a dengue epidemic affected that municipality in the state of Sao Paulo. Eighty percent of the approximately 20,000 people to whom the medicine was distributed on an experimental basis were saved from contracting the disease despite living in risk areas and close to "Aedes aegypti" mosquito breeding sites. "With this compound the disease can last from five to seven days," he specifies. Normally the ailment can be prolonged for two to three weeks.

Medications used in dermatological conditions.
In skin diseases the following drugs may be useful: Arsenicum compositae, Apis mellifica, Apis compositae, Graphites compositae, Hepar sulfur and Thuja.

Compound Arsenicum, 5 sublingual drops every 4-6 hours may be indicated in dry eczema.

Graphites compound at the rate of 5 sublingual drops every 4-6 hours may be indicated in moist eczema.

Medications used as prolactogens.

Within the field of homeopathy there are several drugs used in mammary affections and as prolactogens. In the following, we will give a brief overview of them.

The Dulcamara, whose scientific name is Solanum dulcamara, belongs to the family of the Solanaceae. Other names (vulgar): Royal vine of Judea, sweet solanum, bitter sweet. It contains a glycoalkaloid other than solamine. The sweetness that is noted in the stems after a while becomes sweet, is attributed to the sugar separated from the glycoalkaloid by the hydrolytic action of saliva. The active principles are solamine and dulcamaric acid.

It is slightly narcotic and is used against bronchitis and whooping cough, to combat intestinal colds and soothe rheumatic pains, acts as a depurative in skin diseases. At high doses it produces vomiting and abundant evacuations. Used in chronic blenorrhagia and urethral discharge. For its narcotic effects, without excess, can be tested against insomnia. It seems to affect especially the mucous membranes and has a tendency to establish or discharge both acute and chronic. The patient is disturbed by every change of temperature, from hot to cold, from dry to wet, like catching cold quickly when the body is overheated.

This medicine is also used to treat scaly, suppurative or moist herpes, with vesicles that ooze a yellowish watery liquid; in cases of vulvar herpes, on the glans, scrotum and prepuce, peribuccal and premenstrual herpes. Impetigo with vesicles, cases of lumbago, facial paralysis and upper eyelids produced by exposure to wet cold, scabies with burning puritus that worsens in cold weather, torticollis that appears after exposure to wet cold and urticaria.
The Urtica urens has as scientific name is Fleurya cuneata and belongs to the family Urticáceas. Other names (vulgar): Nettle, cow-itch, west indian nettle. The active ingredient is formic acid. It can be applied in decoction for the retention of urine in children, cases of paralysis and rheumatism and to treat cholera. This plant manifests itself as a powerful hemostatic and the leaves are often used as a topical rubefacient. It is also often indicated when there is profuse secretion of mucous surfaces in cases of enuresis and urticaria and spleen disorders. Antidote to the bad effects of eating oysters. It has also been used in gouty diathesis to promote the elimination of uric acid and if lacteal secretion is absent or in the process of disappearing or suppressed; with breast enlargement.

There are other homeopathic prolactogenic drugs such as Agnus castus,

Asafoetida, Coffea, Ignatia, Lac defloratum, Pulsatilla, Ricinus and Zincum, which are used in the following cases:

Agnus castus: Decrease or disappearance of milk in the puerperium, accentuated sadness and with the fixed idea, often repeated, that she is going to die and that nothing can be done to avoid it: sometimes with a very vague sensation that she is dying, with terrible fear of dying.

Asafoetida: Little or no lacteal secretion in the puerperium: in patients with accentuated hysterical background, with very easy fainting and extremely nervous, with noisy belching and hysterical ballooning.

Coffea: Agalactia in the puerperium or tendency to disappear milk in hyperexcitable, hyperactive patients, with notable hypersensitivity, sensory-sensitive, especially to pain: with accentuated insomnia.

Ignatia: Agalactia or gradual disappearance of milk in the breastfeeding woman, as a consequence of emotional factors (fright, grief, mortification, frustrations, etc.) with depression, involuntary crying, great irritability for consolation and contradiction, very changeable mood, etc.

Lac defloratum: Agalactia or disappearance of milk or suppression of milk, can make milk reappear in 12 to 24 hours. In depressed women who have no desire to see or talk to anyone, and sure that they are going to die soon, but without fear of dying, with headaches, photophobia, intense thirst, constipation and tiredness.

Pulsatilla: Agalactia or gradual disappearance of milk from cold drinking, or complete suppression of breast milk with swelling of the breasts in nursing women who become sad, with very easy and soft crying and improved by consolation, with fear in twilight and darkness, great shyness, great desire for open air, aggravated by heat and absence of thirst.

Ricinus: It has a marked action on the breasts that are in the process of depletion of their milk secretion, increasing it in wet nurses. It is usually accompanied by nausea and vomiting, or abundant and odorless diarrhea.

Zincum: Agalactia or gradual disappearance of milk secretion in patients who are startled by the slightest noise, a very characteristic incessant agitation of the feet and an absolute intolerance to the slightest ingestion of wine.

Use of homeopathic medicine in human immunodeficiency.

AIDS is a relatively recent disease, it is not pessimism, but by the time a really effective allopathic medicine is manufactured to eradicate the human immunodeficiency virus, mutations resistant to such treatment will have already appeared, something that we already see with the current treatments. Through the use of homeopathic Q* potentiation and taking into account the "key" planetary aspects of the star Chiron, it would be feasible to obtain a homeopathic remedy, in a relatively short period of time and without registering the inconveniences that the use of chemotherapeutic agents represents. Through the homeopathic potentiation of the blood of an individual carrying HIV, beyond the ponderable limits, it is possible to create in the virus a condition of insecurity over its habitat, so strong that it would prevent its reproduction and force it to leave the body.

Homeopathic medicines that can be used in stomatological treatments (bellon 2013).

The application of homeopathic treatments is useful in chronic conditions but can be used successfully in acute conditions frequent in our daily practice considered as stomatological emergencies, taking into account those conditions that due to the discomfort they cause to the patient or their possible complications require immediate attention of the professional, among which are mentioned: odontalgia, acute abscesses, cellulitis, pericoronaritis, septic osteitis, stomatitis, hemorrhage, trauma and neuralgia. This document mentions the homeopathic medicines most commonly used in the treatment of stomatological emergencies, identifying their indication, according to the way the individual reacts to a certain disease. This therapy does not replace mechanical procedures, but facilitates the elimination of the acute symptoms present in each condition.

Natural traditional medicine, known internationally as alternative, energetic, naturalist or complementary and holistic medicine, is a reality present throughout the world, forming part of the cultural heritage of each country.

The World Health Organization (WHO) has been promoting the integrated organization of traditional systems of medicine as part of primary health care programs, and has encouraged the study of their potential use as one of the basic pillars on which this care should be based.

Homeopathy is a therapeutic system that uses natural medicines whose objective is to cure according to the laws of healing. It was created by Christian Frederic Hahneman more than 200 years ago and is based on the principle of similarity, an ancient principle proposed by Hippocrates and put into practice by Hahneman, which recognizes the body's ability to heal itself and states that the disease can be cured by substances capable of causing a condition or symptom similar to that of the disease to be treated.

All of them, conveniently prepared, carry stored in their bosom, a certain amount of electromagnetic energy, which acts on the human organism. This medicinal force is called Potency, which is obtained and varies by means of the dynamo-dilutions. There is a vast homeopathic experience in the treatment of chronic conditions, which are described in the classical literature, based on the fact that in the selection of the remedy, the local, general and mental symptoms of the subject are taken into account. However, its usefulness has been proven in acute conditions that are very frequent in stomatological practice.

multiple advantages and benefits with minimal side effects: cost savings and opening of a new line of research and treatment. The objective of this matetrial is to show the possible Homeopathic medicines to be used in the treatment of different stomatological emergencies, taking into account the way each patient suffers from these conditions.

For the application of homeopathic therapy in the treatment of stomatologic emergencies, low or medium potency medicines should be used, with the greatest similarity to the way each individual reacts to a given disease, in other words, the way each individual suffers from the disease should be taken into account.

The following are the most frequent emergencies and the medications indicated for each one of them.

The indicated dose is usually the application of 5 drops sublingually every 15 minutes for 1 hour or until symptoms disappear. After that, the patient is instructed to apply 5 drops sublingually 3 times a day. The patient is instructed to eliminate the treatment when the symptoms disappear. Another form of application of homeopathic medicines is the so-called "Plus Method", which consists of diluting 5 drops of the medicine in half a glass of water. This method is generally indicated in children and in patients sensitive to alcohol.

Odontálgia:

According to Bellon (2013) the most commonly used homeopathic medicines in these conditions we have:

Belladonna: when the patient comes for consultation with right-sided throbbing pain that comes and goes and is aggravated by cold or opening the mouth. The face is red and hot. Mydriasis is evident, the gaze is fixed and the patient is restless and irritable.

Coffea: When the patient presents extreme sensitivity that is relieved with cold water, he/she comes in desperation. E.g.: Acute suppurative pulpitis.

Lachesis: When the patient presents with throbbing pain in the left hemiarch that comes and goes, it can be caused by thermal stimuli (cold), brushing, after eating, chewing, it can also appear before and during menstruation.

Phosphoric magnesia: When the patient presents intense pain that is aggravated by thermal stimulation (cold) and improves with heat. It differs from Coffea in that the patient presents with nervousness and intolerable pain.

Pulsatilla: When the patient comes referring a pain as if they were pulling the nerve that appears in the evening, at bedtime, when clenching teeth, during menstruation, which is aggravated by cold and improves with heat. The patient arrives crying softly.

Staphisagria: When mainly the lower teeth on the right side are affected and it is aggravated by cold, at night, when drinking cold beverages, after eating and during menstruation.

Aranea diadema: When the patient presents violent pain in the maxilla and mandible, when lying down, it intensifies with cold; the patient reports improvement when smoking or when going outdoors.

Coccinela septempuntata: When the patient presents with throbbing pain, with a sensation of coldness, it improves when sleeping. The pain is mainly in the right upper first molar.

Acute abscess, Cellulitis, Periodontal abscess and Pericoronaritis:

In these conditions, the most commonly used drugs are:

Belladonna: When the patient presents with pulsating pain that comes and goes and also refers to a sensation of inflammation (not clinical), this occurs on the right side and redness is also evident in the right hemiface.

Hepar sulfhur: In painful abscesses, very sensitive, with collection of pus that when drained appears mixed with blood. The patient is irritable, violent, the tooth cannot be touched due to hypersensitivity to contact in the affected area.
The abscess shows fluctuating in the area. This medicine is also called homeopathic scalpel.

Silicea: (Similar to Hepar). This medicine is draining, reduces excessive circulation. It is used in acute abscesses with fistulas, in intense fluctuating inflammations. The patient is agitated, restless, irritable, crying, sensation of hair in the mouth.

Lachesis: When there are violent abscesses that do not tolerate contact. Refers to feel heat flares, hypersensitive to contact and heat. Aggravated before menstruation, worse after sleep. Locuaces.

Taréntula cubensis: If the abscesses are of severe evolution, very acute, burning (makes you walk desperately) with hardening of the affected area, pain on contact, rapid prostration and diarrhea.

Myristica sebifera: (avoids the use of the scalpel, like Hepar). It hastens suppuration, short-term drainage in fistulas, traumatic infections, the patient improves in the open air, rapid pulse, restlessness.

Alveolitis and Septic Osteitis:

Nux vomica: when there are tearing pains of the alveolar bone (dry alveolitis), irate, choleric, (may accompany inflammation).

Hepar sulphur: If there is fungal alveolitis with pus, bone suppuration, pain in alveolar tissue, sensitive to contact, improves with heat (fever may occur), the patient is irritated.

Siliceous: When there is presence of fistula by debris or spicules. The patient is restless, agitated and tearful.

Mercurius solubilis: indicated when pain increases at night, with dense saliva, flaccid tongue, jagged, halitosis, thick, abundant saliva.

GUNA:
Secale cormutun: If it presents gangrenous mouth, fetid breath, great bloody suppuration, burning gum-tearing pains.

Lachesis: In gangrenous mouths, foul breath, does not tolerate contact, aggravated before menstruation. Locuaz, bleeding, ulcers that do not tolerate contact.

Mercurius solubilis: If there is foul breath, thick saliva, toothed tongue, aggravated at night, fetidness, tartness on the tongue.

Arnica montana: When it presents foul breath, putrid odor, bleeds easily, does not want to be touched.

Anthracinum: Used alone after not resolving with another. Blackish red bleeding, inflammation, sweetened gums, great fetidness.

GEHA:

Arsenicum album: Burning, pruritic, painful ulcers, restlessness, anxiety of sipping cold water appear.

Cantharis: If it presents vesicles on the mucous membrane of the lips, raw flesh, heat in the mouth similar to Mercurius corrosivus.

Dulcamara: Presence of painful, burning vesicles on the mucosa of the lips, pain with humidity and cold.

Belladonna: If you have painful, burning ulcers on the mucous membranes of the lips, tongue, right cheek, red face, bright eyes.

Natrium Muriaticum: When the mucous membranes of the lips, tongue, cheek are affected, sad, melancholic, resentful, anguished crying.

Rhus tox: In the presence of burning, painful, pruritic gums of the entire oral mucosa, fever and general malaise, great restlessness.

Hemorrhage:

Arnica montana: Effective in hemorrhages of traumatic origin or post-extraction. China: If there is unclotted blood, generalized cold, darkening of vision, noise in the ears, (one of the best hemostatics).

Phosphoro: When they are hemorrhages with predominance of left zone, affectionate, desire for company.

Lachesis: When the hemorrhage is abundant and is related to menstruation or menopause, loquacious.

Secale cornutum: If we observe persistent hemorrhage, black blood, does not tolerate heat, with burning pains and general weakness.

Hanmamelis: If abundant black blood of traumatic origin, followed by rapid prostration.

Facial neuralgia:

Aconitum: When presented on the left side, by exposure to dry and cold wind, with throbbing pain, restlessness, anxiety.

Arsenicum: If you have burning pains, right side, aggravated by cold and light, improved by local heat, fear of dying, anxiety, restlessness.

Belladonna: If it occurs on the right side extending to the ear, appears and disappears at night, aggravated by cold air and movement. Often appears bright red and hot face.

Cedrum: When it affects the right side, appearing every 24 or 48 hours, at the same time. Specific to irritable nervous women.

Stomatitis añosa:

Arsenicum: When symptoms worsen after midnight, metallic taste. The patient is better with heat, restless and exhausted. There is irritable weakness and unquenchable thirst. Burning is relieved by heat. Fear, fright and worry.

Baptisia: If the patient has foul breath and tongue with burning sensation. The patient can only swallow liquid, does not tolerate solid food.
Kreosotum: If it presents putrid odor and bitter taste. Cancer of the tongue and gangrene are the prominent symptoms of the drug.

Mercurius corrosivus: indicated in the loss of teeth with purple, swollen and spongy gums, salivation and bleeding.

Borax: When we observe canker sores on the tongue, cheeks, very painful, bleeding on contact, swollen lips, changing mood, extremely sensitive to noise.

Bibliographic references

1. Agustí, P. 1998. Homeopathy. Ediciones y distribuciones Mateos, pp. 16-17.

2. Almunia, A.; Estrada, M. and Pérez, F. 1998. Homeopathy. Homeopathic therapeutics. Cuban Rev. of Integral Medicine. 13(4):369-371.

3. Alonso-Andicoberry C, García-Peña FJ, Ortega-Mora LM. Epidemiology, diagnosis and control of bovine leptospirosis. Investig Agr Prod Sanid Anim 2001;16:205-25.

4. Alvarez, M.A.; Cervantes, L.P.; Rosas, D.; Vazquez, C. and. Garcia, F.S (2005). Retrospective study of bovine Leptospirosis seroprevalence in Mexico considering ecological regions. Rev. Cub. Med. Trop., 57 (1): 28-31.

5. Amaral MS. Holistic Dentistry. Nature, teeth and health. Sao Paulo: Edit Jornalistica Lido; 1994.

6. Amaral S M. Holistic dentistry. Sao Paulo: Edit Mitos; 1994.

7. Ancarola, R. 1996. Homeopathic treatment of the chronically ill. Madrid. Spain. (Editorial) pp. 19-20.

8. Angeleri A., Lucca D. S. Responsibility and health...Arguments to sterilize your pet. Rev.World Society for the protection of anímáis, pp 5 - 8. 2007.

9. Barros, St. and Pasteur, J. 1992. Homeopathy, Land Medicine. 3rd ed. Universidad Central de Venezuela. Caracas. Ediciones de la Biblioteca, p. 16.

10. Berthier, D. 1991. Guía práctica de la Homeopatía para todos. Indigo, Barcelona, Spain.

11. Berdasquera D., Rodríguez I., Obregón A. M., Fernández C., Segura R., Bustabad E., Sánchez C.M. Outbreak of human Leptospirosis in Guantánamo province: Reflections of an Epidemic. Pedro Kourí" Institute of Tropical Medicine. Rev. Cubana Med. Trop; 59(1). 2006.

12. Berdasquera, D.C.; Rodríguez, Islay, G.; Miralles, F.A.; Obregón, Ana, M.; Fernández, Carmen, M. (2006). Human leptospirosis in Guantanamo province: reflections of an epidemic. Juventud Rebelde newspaper. Available at URL:

http://www.juventudrebelde.cu/secciones/perfiles/guantanamo.html.
[Accessed May 18, 2008],

13. Bertossi, E. 1993. Homeopathy and Preventive Medicine. Homeopathy and Nature. 3:17-18.

14. BIODENT. Nosodes. [online]. Neurofocal dentistry (2002). Available at: http://www.odontoloqianeurofocal.com/nosodes.htm

15. Bofill, P.; Rivas, A.; Ramirez, W.; Montañez, J.; Martinez, A.; Quincoses, T.; Reinaldo, L. and Fustes, E. 1988. Bacterial diseases. In su: Manual of infectious diseases. Volume I. Havana. Ediciones ISCAH. pp. 3-59.

16. Brand, R. 1994. Adream on the origin of action of homeopathic remedies. British Homeopathic Journal. 44(6):141-143.

17. Briones, S.F. 1990. Manual of Homeopathic Veterinary Medicine. Theory and Practice of the application of Homeopathy in Veterinary Medicine. Santiago de Chile. Hochstetler. LTDA.

18. Briones, S.F. 1996. Manual of Homeopathic Veterinary Medicine. Theory and practice of the application of homeopathy in veterinary medicine. 2nd ed. Santiago de Chile. De Hochstetler Ltda. pp. 50-53.

19. Briones, S.F. Homeopathic treatment trial of subclinical mastitis in dairy cattle [online]. Homeopathy in Animal Production (2001). Available at:http://members.Trؚpod.com/~Flavؚo.Brؚones/pollos.htm.

20. Briones, S.F. Study of the effect of *Calcárea carbónica* 50 M, 30a and *Calcárea fosfórica* 50 M, 3a, on weight gain in pigs [online]. Homeopathy in Animal Production (1987). Available at: http://members.Trؚpod.com/~Flavؚo.Brؚones/pollos.htm.

21. Callejo, R.F . Homeopathy [online]. My point of view (2000). Available at: http://web.madhtel.es/personales3/rfcalleio/punto.htm

22. Calvinho, L.F. 1999. Efficacy and elimination time in milk of penetamate hydrochloride in clinical mastitis caused by *Streptococcus*. Preliminary report. Proceedings of the National Congress on Milk Quality and Mastitis. Río Cuarto.

23. Campos H. A. Head of Todo para tu mascota, Mexico D.F. 2006. Available at http://www.veterinaria.org/ajfa/nota05.htm . Accessed April 2007.

24. Carneiro I. Homeopathy. Popular orientation. IV ed. Sao Paulo: Brazil; 1993.

25. Carolina Maria. Co-founder of Animal Homeopathy/Veterinary

Homeopathy in Bogotá. Available at: javascript: void (o) i./mascotas/guiasapoyo/. 2007. Accessed February 2008.

26. Cass, L. and Chein, E. Benefits of homeopathic (HGH) [online] (1999). Available at: http:

//www.reiuvin.com/spanish/HGH%20v%20homeopatia.htm

27. Celorio, Silvia M. 1999. Homeopathy: a biophysical point of view. Conference. Faculty of Medical Sciences. Cienfuegos. Cuba.

28. Cepero O., Bonet J. Influence of certain climatological variables on the incidence rate of Leptospirosis in humans and behavior of this entity in the province of Villa Clara in the period 1997-2002. Paper presented at the Student Forum. UCLV. 2008.

29. Charanon P. Memento homeopathique D" urgence Cinquine. Moscow Edit Dangles; 1988: 71.

30. Chavez, J. 1996. How a producer who produces milk with more than 500 000 somatic cells and/or high bacterial counts should act. Proceedings of the National Congress on Milk Quality and Mastitis. Río Cuarto, pp. 67-68.

31. Chin J. The control of communicable diseases. Washington DC: PAHO. (581): 409-12. 2001.

32. Chuchini, U.N. and Mirón, N.l. 1987. Electrón acupunture for serous mastitis in cows. Vet. Bull. 57(11):45-46.

33. Cummings, S. 1991. Practical Guide to Homeopathic Medicine. Madrid, Spain. Ediciones EDAF, S.A. pp. 30-35.

34. De Medio, H. 1997. Introduction to Homeopathic Veterinary Medicine. Buenos Aires, Argentina. Ed. Albatros.

35. Terminological dictionary of medical sciences. XI ed. Edit Científico Técnica; Havana; 1984.

36. Dudgeon, R.E y Jain, B. 1997. Lectures on the Theory & Practice of Homoeopathy, Publishers (P) Ltd, Lecture VI, Isopathy. pp. 141 - 175.

37. Dulcetti O. Homeopathy in dentistry. Riberao Preto: IMFL; 1983:113. 3. Guajardo B.G. How Homeopathy has survived. La Homeopatía de México 2000; 69 (604): 18-21.

38. Dyson, F. 1971. Energy in the Universe Scunt. Ámsterdam. p. 51.

39. Edwards, J. 1995. The Homeopathic treatment of pain anímáis. British Homeopathic Journal. 45(3):52-55.

40. Epstein, P.R.; Pena, O.C. y Racedo, J.B. (1995). Climate and disease in

Colombia. Lancet; 346:1243-1244.

41. Errecalde, J.O. 1996. Use of new antibiotics and other drugs to eliminate infections during lactation and dry period. Proceedings of the National Congress on Milk Quality and Mastitis. Río Cuarto. Conf. 15.

42. Everald C. D., Edwards C. N., Everald J. D. A. Twelve years study of Leptospirosis on Barbados. Eur. S. Epideniel. 11(3): 311 -320. 1995.

43. Faine S, Adler B, Bolín C, Perolat P. Leptospira and leptospirosis, 2nd ed. Melbourne:MediSciÓ; 2000.

44. Feresu S.B., Bolín C.A., Korver H., Van-de-Kemp H. Identification of Leptospires of the pomona and grippotyphosa serogroups isolated from cattle in Zimbabwe. Res. Vet. Sci. 59(1): 92-94. 1995.

45. Fernandez J. 1998. Veterinary Homeopathy. In. Rev. ADDA. Barcelona, Spain. Ediciones ADDA. 18: 17-20. March.

46. Ferrara, L.; Scaramelli, A.M. and Troya, H.R. 1998. Prevalence of subclinical bovine mastitis in Venezuela and evaluation of the California test for mastitis. Proceedings of the Pan-American Congress on Mastitis Control and Milk Quality. Merida, Yucatan, Mexico, p. 46.

47. Finch, J.M.; Winter, A.; Walton, A.W. and Leigh, J.A. Further studies on the efficacy of a live vaccine against mastitis caused by *Streptococcus uberis* [en línea] Vaccine 15(10):1138-43 (1997). Disponible en: http://www.ncbi.nlm.nih.qov/entrez/querv.fcqi?cmd=Retrieve&db=PubMed&list ui ds=9269059&dopt=Abstrac

48. Flores, A. and Flores, C. What is homeopathy? [online] (1999). Available at: http://www.homeopatia.cib.net.htm

49. Fox, L.K. and Gay, J.M. 1993. Contagious mastitis. Veterinary Clinics of North America: Food Animal Practice 9:475-487.

50. Fuentes, R. 1996. Plant species in Cuba used in the preparation of homeopathic medicines. Rev. Cubana de Plantas Medicinales 1(3):3-8. Sept-Dec.

51. Fustes, E. 1991. Mastitis, some aspects of its control. Revista popular de divulgación agropecuaria de Cuba 1:45-47.

52. Garcia C. Flomeopatíaovinay caprina. http://www.capraispana.com/libros/eco/portasdarco.jpg. . 2007. Accessed March 2008.

53. García C. and Félix Tratamiento antiparasitario en ganadería ecológica.

http://www.capraispana.com/libros/eco/portasdarco.jpg. . 2007. Retrieved March 2008.

54. García Ch., Paz R., Borroto P. Geoepidemiology of human Leptospirosis in Cuba. Rev. Cubana de Fligiene y Epidemiología; 34(1): 15-22. 1996.

55. Gasque, R. and Blanco, M.A. Bovine mastitis [cd-room]. In: Zootecnia en bovinos productores de leche [Mexico City]: UNAM. 2001. pp. 155-171.

56. Gerritson M.J., Koopmans, M.J., Olyhock, T. Effect of streptommycin treatment on the sheddind of and the serologic responses to L. interrogans serovar hardjo subtype hardjobovis in experimentally infected cows. Vet. Microbiol. 38(1-2): 129-135. 1993.

57. Golden, I. Flomeopathic Desease Prevention. [online]. 1999. Available at: http://www.qolden/homeophatic.htm.

58. Gonzalez J.A., Tamayo S., Machado A. Leptospirosis. Editorial CIDA. Havana, pp. 22-31. 1990.

59. González J. A., Machado A. Some aspects on Leptospirosis in Villa Clara province. IV National Meeting on Leptospirosis. Santa Clara. 1993.

60. González Y. Behavior of the Serological and Epizootiological analysis of Leptospirosis in the year 2000-2005 in Villa Clara. Work presented at the IMV Villa Clara Base Forum. 2006.

61. Gonzalez, N.R. 1996. The New York State Mastitis Control Program. United States of America. Proceedings of the National Congress on Milk Quality and Mastitis. Río Cuarto, pp. 9-19.

62. Gordon, A. 1981. Homeopathy. EDAF, Madrid, Spain, pp. 12-24. Q2.

63. Grosso, A. 1987. Homeopathic Veterinary Medicine Pages. 2nd ed. Buenos Aires, Argentina. El Ateneo.

64. Guajardo, B. 1997. Comparative Study of Homeopathic and Allopathic Treatments of bovine subclinical mastitis. Research Work. Veterinary Science Research Institute. UABC. Mexico.

65. Guajardo, G. 1994. Seminar on Pharmacology of Homeopathic medicines. "New Horizons in Veterinary Therapeutics". U.N.A.M., Mexico D. F. pp. 55 -56.

66. Guajardo, G. 1998. On the popularization of Homeopathy. Homeopathy in Mexico. Vol. 67 July-August (595) pp. 120-125.

67. Guillén, J. 1994. Active Information Bulletin. Drug Information Center. Havana, Cuba. 18:2-18.

68. Gutiérrez M. Conference at the Scientific Society of Veterinary Clinics. VMI. June 2010.

69. Hahneman S. Homoeopathy, the newest edition of the organon of medicine. Caracas: Univ Central de Venezuela. Edit de la Biblioteca; 1983.

70. Hahnemann, S. 1999. Organon of Medicine. Reprinted edition. Buenos Aires. Editorial Lito. pp. 50-60.

71. Hillerton, J.E. 1996. Control of mastitis. In: Progress in Dairy Science. Wallingford, Oxon, UK. Edited by C.J.C. Phillips, CAB International, pp. 171-190.

72. Hogan, J.S. and Smith, K.L. Risk factors associated with environmental mastitis [en línea] (1998). National Mastitis Council Annual Meeting Proceedings. p. Disponible at:http://www.nmconline.org/articles/riskfactors.htm

73. Homan, Jane and Wattiaux, M. Mastitis [cd-room]. In: Dairy Technical Guides: Lactation and Milking [Wisconsin]: Babcock Institute for International Research and Development for the Dairy Industry. University of Wisconsin. 1999. pp. 61-76.

74. Hubener S. Infectious diseases of domestic animals III Edition. Editorial Acribia. Spain, pp.112- 120. 1996.

75. Hunter, F.E. 1996. My cat is driving me crazy! British Homeopathic Journal. 46(5): 118.

76. I.B.E.H.E. 1997. Homeopathy, Principles, Doctrine and Pharmacy. 2nd edition, Sao Paulo, Brazil. Ed. Mythos. pp. 110-115.

77. Leptospirosis Report. Provincial Center of Hygiene and Epidemiology. Villa Clara. 2006.

78. Instituí Pasteur. Biological Diagnosis. Leptospirosis-Lime Disease. Paris:lnstitut Pasteur; 2000.

79. Jayasuriya, A. 1988. Clinical Homeophatic. B. Join Publishers. New Delhi, India, pp. 1-2; 3-10; 25-32; 118; 363; 583.

80. Kastli, P. 1967. Definition of Mastitis. A Bull. Int. Dairy Fed. Part. 11:1.

81. Kent JT. Lessons in Homeopathic Materia Medica. 3rd ed: B Jain Publishers Put, Ltd; (205-208). New Delhi 1994

82. Lago D, Rodríguez J. Scientific information in Homeopathy . Rev Summary 2001; 14(1):10-21

83. Landeros, M. 1996. Homeopathy and its application in Veterinary

Medicine. Homeopathic Gazette 1(1):8-10.

84. Lazo L. Lecture of the Veterinary Preventive Medicine Diploma of the Veterinary Clinic specialty. Faculty of Agricultural Sciences. UCLV. June 2009.

85. Leigh, J.A. Vaccines against bovine mastitis due to *Streptococcus uberis* current status and future prospects [en línea], Adv. Exp. Med. Biol. 480:307-311 (2000). Disponible en: http://www.ncbi.nlm.nih.qov/entrez/querv.fcqi?cmd=Retrieve&db=PubMe b&list ui ds=10959438&dopt=Abstract

86. Lenderman, J. 1996. Homeopathy in the Wild: Ranger, the Harbour Seal. British Homeopathic Journal. México 46(1): 15-16.

87. Lessele BC. A text book of dental: Homeopathy. Edit. Daniel Comp LTD. Londres: 1995

88. Levett P.N. Leptospirosis. Clin Microbiol Rev. 14(2): 296-326. 2001.

89. Liebe, A. and Scham, S.D. 1998. Growth factors in milk: Interrelation ships with somatic cell count. J. Dairy Res. 65(1):93-100.

90. Linares F. Homeopathic Vademecum. Labiofam. Cienfuegos. 2004.

91. Little, D. Nosodes in Homeopathy [online] Case Management (1999). Available at: http://www.simillimun.com/thelittlelibrarv/casemanaqe

92. Lockie, A. and Geldir, N. 1995. Routes for the use of homeopathic medicines. Complete Guide to Homeopathy. USA. pp. 53.

93. Loor, J.J.; Jones, G.M. and Bailey, T.L. Basics of mastitis development [online]. Virginia Polytechnic Institute and University (1999). Blacksburg. Available from: http://www.dasc.vt.edu/jones/UnderstandinqMastitis(spanish).htm

94. López P.M., Ortega S.C., Atilano L., De la Peña M.A. Detection of antibodies against Leptospira Interrogans in equines dedicated to the production of hyperimmune sera. Veterinaria. Mexico. 29(2); 173-179.1998.

95. López R. "Homeopathy and Animal Health". Homeopatía de México No 606 P. 99 Vol. 69 May - June 2000.

96. Luis, M.P. Homeopathy [online] (2003). Available at: http://www.saludnatural.net/Homeo.htm

97. Luna-Álvarez M.A., Moles-Cervantes L.P., Gavaldón-Rosas D. Nava-Vázquez C. and Salazar-García F. Retrospective study of bovine

leptospirosis seroprevalence in Mexico considering ecological regions. Rev. Cub. Med. Trop., 57 (1): 28- 31. 2005.

98. Machado A. Second International Meeting on Leptospirosis. CIDA, Havana, 1997.

99. Machado A. Situation of Leptospirosis in Villa Clara Province. Annual Technical Meeting. IMV Villa Clara. February 10, 2010.

100. Magill A.J. Fever in returned travrler. Infecí. Dis. Clin. North Am. 12(2): 445-469. 1998.

101. Malakhov Y. A., Alejin J. Leptospirosis of animals. Editorial Ciencias Médicas. Havana, p. 435. 2007.

102. Manual of Homeopathic Pharmacy Technical Standards . 1997. Havana, Cuba. pp. 5-32.

103. Martín R. Guantánamo Province. Juventud Rebelde newspaper. Available at: http://www.juventudrebelde.cu/secciones/perfiles/guantanamo.html. Cited July 18, 2006.

104. Martínez R., Álvarez A.M. Efficacy and safety of a vaccine against human Leptospirosis in Cuba. Rev Panam Salud Publica. 15(4): 249-55. 2004.

105. Martínez R., Armesto M. Evaluation of the effectiveness of a new vaccine against Human Leptospirosis: Rev. Panam. de Salud Pública. (8):385-92. 2000.

106. Martínez R., Pérez A., Quiñones M.C., Cruz R., Álvarez A.M., Armesto M. Efficacy and safety of a vaccine against human Leptospirosis in Cuba. Rev Panam Public Health. 15(4):249-55. 2004.

107. Martínez, Elsa; Ponce, P.; Ginorio, Caridad; López, María G. and Morales, Caridad. 1992. Control of the hygienic quality of milk: a necessary condition from the cow to the consumer. Memorias del Encuentro-Taller sobre control de la calidad de la leche y derivados lácteos. Cuba. pp. 184- 207.

108. Martínez, J. 1979. Homeopathic pharmacy. Pharmaceutical Doctrine and Technique. Spain. Ed. Albatros.

109. Martínez, J. 1990. Homeopathic Pharmacy. Spain. Ed. Albatros. pp. 13- 22.

110. Masón R.J., Fleming P.J., Smythe L.D., Dohnt M.F., Norris M.A., Symonds M.L. Leptospira interrogans antibodies in feral pig from New South Wales. J. Wildl. Dis. 34(4): 738-743.1998.

111. Medina D, M; Jaramillo C, G; Borja C, G. (1998). Leptospirosis in the coastal region of Ecuador: an announced epizootic. Rev. CIEZT; 3(2):45-55.

112. Merck. The Merck manual of veterinary medicine eighth edition in Spanish. Editorial Océano. Barcelona Spain pp. 616 and 617. 2005.

113. Mermel L.A. Fluman and animal leptospirosis. J. Emerg. Med. 16(6): 97851-6. 1998.

114. Miguel Ángel Luna Álvarez and others .REV CUBANA MED TROP 2005;57(1):28- 31

115. Montesino, C.V. and Arocha, B.O.E. (2001). Behavior of human Leptospirosis. Rev. Cub. Enf. v.17 n.3 Ciudad de la Habana Sep.-Dec. 2001. Available at URL: www.scielo.sld.cu/scielo.php? [Accessed March 4, 2008],

116. Morfin, Lilian and Camacho , M. 1990. Weight increase in piglets through the administration of a homeopathic compound. Homeopathy in Mexico, pp. 2-10.

117. Morfin, Lilian. Application of Homeopathy in Veterinary Medicine to combat Mastitis [online] (2002). Available at: http://www.homeoorq.mx/mastitis.htm.

118. Morfin, Lilian. Homeopathy for cows! [online]. Research and Development. Science and Technology Journalism (November 1999). Available at: http://www.invdes.com.mx/suplemento/anteriores/noviembre1999/htm.

119. Morin, D.E. and Hurley, W.L. Mastitis. Lesson B. [en línea]. Lactation Biology. ANSCI 308. University of Illinois (1994). Urbana-Champaign. Disponible en:http://classes.aces.uiuc.edu/AnSci308/mastjtjsb.htm

120. Muratas, J. 1990. Lessons in Homeopathy. 2nd ed. Austrian Academy of Homeopathy Publishing House, pp. 67-78.

121. National Mastitis Council. 1995. Mastitis Control in Dairy Herds. Cap. 9:229-277.

122. NC 118:01. Milk. California test for diagnosis of mastitis. July 2001.

123. NC 78-25:86. Milk and milk products: "Sampling". July 1986.

124. NC ISO 13366-1:97. Milk. Enumeration of somatic cells. Microscopic method. October 1997.

125. Nickerson, S.C. 1998. Strategies to control mastitis. Proceedings of the

Pan-American Congress on Mastitis Control and Milk Quality. Merida, Yucatan, Mexico, p. 5.

126. Noguera, E. The best way to control bovine mastitis [online]. FONAIAP-CIAE. Ministry of Science and Technology. National Institute of Agricultural Research (1999).   Venezuela. Available   at: http://www.fona¡ap.qov.ve/publica/d¡vulqa/fd59/mast¡t¡s.html.

127. Novoa, R.M.; Armenteros, Mabelín; Abeledo, María Antonia; Casanovas, E.; Valera, R. and Pulido, J.L. 2002. Epizootiological and economic evaluation of bovine mastitis in specialized dairy herds in Cienfuegos province. XVIII Pan-American Congress of Veterinary Sciences. Havana. Havana. November.

128. O'Byrne, A. Course XII. Biotherapy [online]. Nosodetherapy. Sarcodeterapia.   (2003)   Colombia.   Available   at: http://members.tripod.com/cmbick0/id27.htm

129. Obregón A.M., Fernández C., Rodríguez I., Rodríguez J., Fernández N. Enrique G. Importance of microbiological confirmation in an outbreak of human Leptospirosis in the city of Villa Clara. Rev. Cubana Med. Trop. 55(2). 2003. Available en: http://scielo.sld.cu/scielo.php?pid=S0375-07602003000200006&script=sci_arttext.

130. Obregón AM, Fernández C, Rodríguez I, Rodríguez J, Fernández N, Enrique G. (2003). Importance of microbiological confirmation in an outbreak of human Leptospirosis in the city of Villa Clara. Rev Cubana Med Trop 2003; 55(2).

131. Ogata, A. and Nagahata, H. Intramammary application of ozone therapy to acute clinical mastitis in dairy cows [en línea], J. Vet. Med. Sci. 62(7):681-684 (2000). Disponible en: http://www.ncb¡.nlm.n¡h.qov/entrez/querv.fcq¡?cmd=Retrieve&db=PubMed&l¡st u¡ ds=10945283&dopt=Abstract

132. Oliva R., Infante J. F., González M., Pérez V., Sifontes S. Pathologic clinical characterization of leptospirosis in a golden sirion hamster model. Arch. Med. Res. 25 (2): p. 165-170. 1994.

133. WHO. The control of communicable diseases. Seventeenth edition. Scientific-Technical Publications. PAHO. N ^{0} 581.pp. 50-54. 2001.

134. WHO.PAHO. World Health Organization Strategy on Natural and Traditional   Medicine   2002-

2005.http://www.16deabril.sld.cu/rev/206/mnt.html. Alternative Medicine.

135. Osés, R (2004): "Meteorological series of Villa Clara and other provinces", Thesis for the category of Master in Applied Mathematics, UCLV, 2004.

136. Osés, R. (2008). Personal communications. Master of Science. Researcher of the Provincial Meteorological Center (CMP). Villa Clara. Cuba.

137. Osés, R.R. (2004). Meteorological series of Villa Clara and other provinces;

138. Palsule S G. Dentistry and Homoeopathy .New Delhi; B. Jain Publishers; 1997.

139. Paschero, T.P. 1999. Homeopathy. 4th ed. Buenos Aires, Argentina. Editorial El Ateneo, pp 90-93.

140. Pecker, Jackeline 1990. Birds and Homeopathy. Homeopathy in Mexico. Editorial Armate, pp. 11-13:26.

141. Peeler, E.; Green, M.; Fitzpatrick, J.; Morgan, K. and Green, L. 2000. Risk factors associated with clinical mastitis in low somatic cell count british dairy herds. J. Dairy Sci. 83(11):2464-2472, november.

142. Pereira, S. Homeopathic medicines [online]. First Argentine portal of unicist homeopathy and alternative therapy (2000). Available at: http://www.unicista.com/medicamentos.htm

143. Pérez, A.; Morfin, Lilian and Camacho, M. 1998. Preliminary evaluation of a biotherapeutic in the treatment of subclinical mastitis in dairy cattle. XVI Pan-American Congress of Veterinary Sciences, 9-13 Nov. Santa Cruz de la Sierra, Bolivia. p. 143.

144. Granma Newspaper   . 1997. Homeopathy also in animals. Havana.

145. Philpot, W.N. Importance of somatic cell count and factors affecting it [online]. III National Congress on Mastitis Control and Milk Quality. Léon, Gto.   Mexico   (June   2001).   Available   at: http://www.cnmweb.bizland.com/publicaciones/DrPhilpot2.PDF

146. Philpot, W.N. 1996. Milk Quality and Mastitis. Dissertation delivered at the First Latin American Dairy Production and Industry Exhibition: Dairy World. Argentina, p. 1.

147. Philpot, W.N. 2000. Strategies for controlling mastitis. Dissertation delivered at the Vil Congreso Panamericano de la Leche. FEPALE. Havana. Havana. Cuba.

148. Philpot, W.N. and Nickerson, S.C. 1993. Mastitis: The counterattack   .

A strategy for combating mastitis. Published by Babson Bros. Co.

149. Prescott, J.F. and Baggot, J.D. 1993. Antimicrobial therapy in medicine veterinary. Blackwell Scientific Publications. Boston, Massachusetts.

150. RESUMED 2001; 14(1):5-9.PDF Format. Edit Homeopathy Homeopathy as a therapeutic strategy.

151. RESUMED 2001; 14(1): 3-4. PDF format. Edit Homeopathy scientific-technical information.

152. Reverón G.M. Homeopathy as a therapeutic strategy. Rev Resumen.2001; 14(1):5-9

153. Riverón, Mayra.   1997. Five questions about Homeopathy. Rev. Cubana de Medicina Integral. Havana. 13(3).

154. Robinson, R. 1996. The nature cure clinic. British Homeopathic Journal. 46(5):111-113.

155. Ryser, L. 1998. Microorganisms of importance in raw milk. Proceedings of the Pan-American Congress on Mastitis and Milk Quality. Mexico.

156. Sánchez PO: Lectures on Homeopathy in Cuba. Homeopathic Medical Association. Tenerife, Canary Islands; 1999.

157. Sánchez, Josefina. 1994. International Seminar on Homeopathic Experimentation. Havana, Cuba.

158. Schwabe, W. 1995. Homeopathic Pharmacopoeia. 2nd ed. in English. Leipzig. Argentina.

159. Sears, P.M. 1990. Mastitis-causing organisms: Diagnosis, source and factors related to their control. Quality milk Newsletler, N.Y. State Mast. Control Prog. 6:3.

160. Silva, Enedina. 1994. Homeopatía Veterinaria, MVZE, pp. 1045-1049, Mexico.

161. Silva, Enedina. 1998. Veterinary Homeopathy. Trials in slaughter animals. México. D.F.

162. Smith, K.L. and Hogan, J.S. 1995. Epidemiology of mastitis. Proceedings of the [3rd] IDF International Mastitis Seminar. Book II. Tel Aviv, Israel. S6:3-12.

163. Solórzano del Río, H. Homeopathy and some of its fundamentals [online]. Terapia Bioquímica Natural (2003). Guadalajara. México. Available at: http://www.hector.solorzano.com/artículos/

164. Speight, P. 1995. Homeopathy at your fingertips. A practical course, Ira.

ed. in Spanish. Editorial Panorama. Mexico.

165. Suarez, R. 1989. Practical Guide to Homeopathic Pharmacopoeia. Buenos Aires. Argentina. Ed. Héctor A. Macchi.

166. Sumano, H.; Brumbaugh, G.W. and Mateos, Gabriela. 1996. Pharmacological basis for the treatment of bovine mastitis. Vet. Mex. 27(1):63-82.

167. Taubin, P. 1959. The vital energy. Homeopathy 26(264):111.

168. Tetau, M. 1998. New theoretical and practical considerations on diluted and dynamized organotherapy. France. Ed. Maloine.

169. Tomazella, J.A. 1995. Treatment of sub clinical mastitis of dairy cattle with milk isotherapic and other homeopathic medicines. Preliminary study. Conchas, Brazil. 55 Panamerican Homeopathic Medical Congress. La Habana. Cuba.

170. Torrijos, G. 1993. Effects of treatments with homeopathic medicines and one with antibiotic against chronic respiratory diseases in birds. Chair of Bromatology of the Facultad de Estudios Superiores, UNAM. Mexico.

171. Valera, R.; Linares, F.; Novoa, R.; Caballero, C. and Casanovas, E. 2002. Homeopathic therapy of bovine subclinical mastitis. XVIII Pan-American Congress of Veterinary Sciences. Havana.

172. Vithoukas, G. 1989. Homeophaty in traditional medicine and health care coverage. World Health Organization, Geneva.

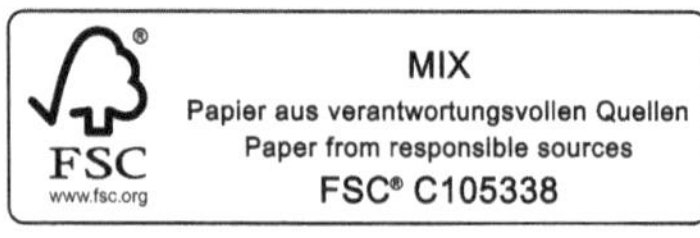

Printed by Books on Demand GmbH, Norderstedt / Germany